ACTUALIZED RECOVERY®

IT'S NOT ABOUT 12-STEPS

RECOVERY IS A BRAIN THING

DAVE KENNEY & SUSAN KENNEY

First published by Ultimate World Publishing 2024

ISBN

Paperback: 978-1-923123-64-9
Ebook: 978-1-923123-65-6

Cover design: Ultimate World Publishing
Layout and typesetting: Ultimate World Publishing
Editor: TBC
Cover image license: MrArtHit-Shutterstock.com

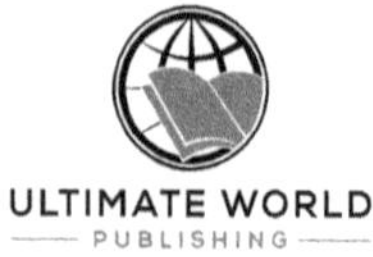

Ultimate World Publishing
Diamond Creek,
Victoria Australia 3089
www.writeabook.com.au

ACTUALIZED RECOVERY®

The Brain-First Approach to Lasting Recovery

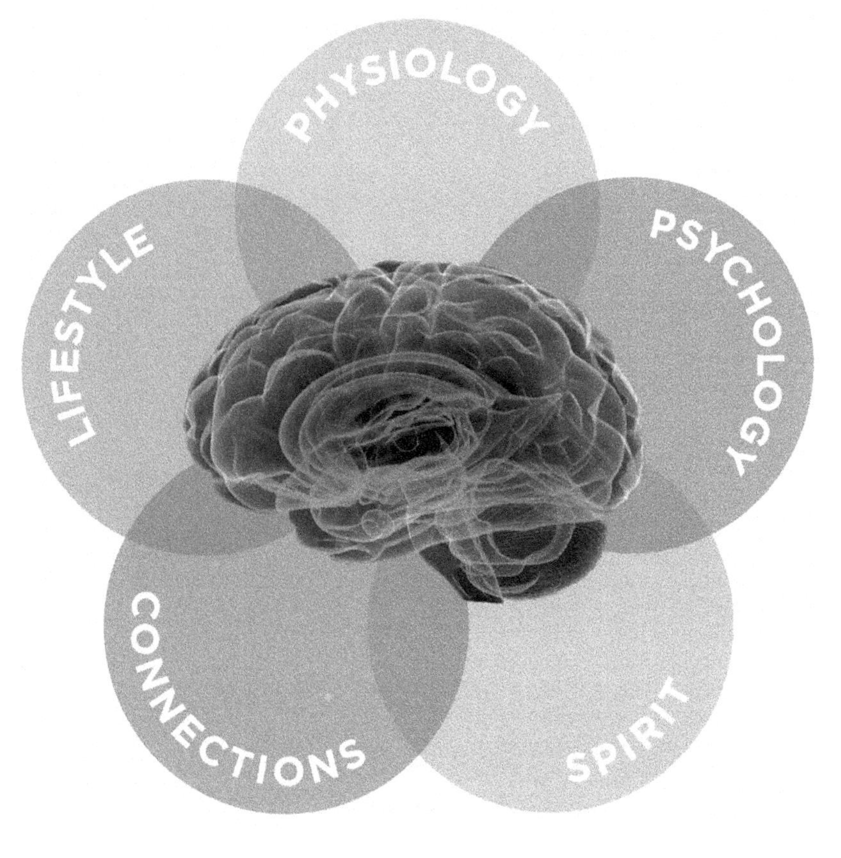

Endorsements

"Finally! A book that gets to the underlying root of WHY people become addicted to harmful substances and the foundational piece that's missing from most recovery programs—the brain!

The brain-first approach in *Actualized Recovery* is a game-changer that has the potential to help so many people overcome addiction."

- Daniel Amen, MD
Double Board-Certified Psychiatrist
World renowned Neuro-Psychiatrist
Nine-Time New York Times Best-Selling Author

"*Actualized Recovery* is undoubtedly one of the most powerful books on overcoming addiction and trauma that I have ever encountered. It presents a proven roadmap, leading readers from the depths of despair to a state of peaceful wellbeing and happiness. The innovative methodology, especially the brain-first approach, establishes a new benchmark in the field of addiction and recovery. This work is a game-changer, empowering individuals to overcome any addiction or behavioral challenge with dignity and grace. It is a truly remarkable and indispensable read for practitioners and anyone seeking a path to living a heroic comeback story."

- Giovanni Marsico, Founder/CEO, Archangel
2x EMMY® Award-Winning Producer

"As a physician with a focus on addiction treatment, I've encountered numerous methodologies and theories on recovery, but *Actualized Recovery*, by Dave Kenney & Susan Kenney, stands out for its revolutionary brain-first approach. This book brilliantly navigates the complexities of addiction recovery, emphasizing the critical role of brain health and functionality. The authors adeptly use the metaphor of the brain as a grand orchestra to illustrate how various brain functions collaborate to influence our thoughts, behaviors, and recovery processes. What I find most compelling is the book's holistic integration of neuroscience, psychology, and lifestyle interventions, offering readers a comprehensive pathway to understanding and overcoming addiction. The treatments and therapies outlined are not only evidence-based but also actionable and deeply resonant with my professional experiences. I highly recommend 'Actualized Recovery' to anyone seeking a profound, sustainable journey towards healing and well-being. This book is a must-read for individuals navigating the challenges of addiction, as well as for professionals in the field. It's a testament to the power of understanding and optimizing our brains to achieve lasting Recovery."

- Dr. Mark Leeds, D.O.
The Rehab Podcast

"Finally! The book *Actualized Recovery* addresses the root understanding of addiction and is a must-read for anyone looking for a solution that makes sense when it comes to behavioral and substance addiction beyond the rooms of 12-Step programs. This book is not just insightful, but it is also written with empathy and care and drives the conversation to "Brain Health," which is a much-missed part of the recovery narrative. Consider a new narrative that connects the dots between body, mind, spirit, and emotions to call forth a holistic blueprint for Recovery.

Dave and Susan Kenney will spark hope, curiosity, and light in the lives of those who read it and those they know who want to win the battle of addiction. It is an honor to take this journey with the authors to help those who struggle ultimately to gain personal freedom, connect with a supportive community, or guide others through tough times as a vocation.

This amazing book aims to provide hope, ignite curiosity, promote learning, and spread light to those struggling and seeking a solution that makes sense. It ignites the spark for others who care about someone who is having challenges and for those who feel frustrated and dismissed by an old paradigm that does not address the causes of behavioral and substance addiction. Additionally, the book is for people who want to learn the evidence-based connection between the brain and behaviors, to gain personal freedom, a sense of hope in action, and to change their lives.

If you are looking for a community to feel supported and uplifted and have the deep desire and calling to guide others through tough times as a vocation, this book provides a "Live Blueprint" full of valuable insights and guidance. For many of us who have been down the pathway of Recovery, this would have been our "wish list" book for living."

- Pat Baccili, PhD
The Dr. Pat Show, and The Transformational Network

"Susan and Dave provide a much-needed update to the antiquated field of addiction treatment. They understand the most crucial aspect of addiction: that it is a symptom of underlying suffering. This concise book introduces people to the range of modern and holistic methods that inspire genuine hope for the reader."

- Daniel Hochman, M.D., Psychiatrist
Creator of Self Recovery:
The Online Addiction Recovery Program

"Susan and Dave Kenney nailed it! Their Brain First approach is a refreshing update for the addiction/recovery community.

Oftentimes, patients are entering treatment, and they have tried multiple avenues to become clean and sober, and they have been unsuccessful, or they have succeeded, but they are still looking for more answers. There's a realization that the substances and/ or behaviors are just a "band-aid over a bullet wound." This book is the response people are looking for.

As a person who was introduced to the world of addiction and recovery (at birth) and continues to work with others as a clinician in the recovery community, this book is a much-needed update on where it all begins— the brain.

With an easy-to-read, detailed way to help others understand how the brain works, I look forward to witnessing how *Actualized Recovery* is received by the addiction/recovery community. It's exciting to take advantage of the discovered science of the brain and put it into action.

Bravo to the Kenney's!"

- Mary Thompson, MA, LPC, LISAC Clinician

"What a treasure! Dave and Susan's extraordinary book is the real thing. It is based on science yet written in a language that everyone can understand. It is replete with real stories that are easy to relate to. It is full of hope, of real tools and so incredibly compelling.

It should be compulsory reading in college but short of that, anyone who has ever struggled with destructive behaviors or anyone who wants to help a loved one in trouble should read it. Wouldn't that be everyone?"

- Helene Flageole MD, MSc, FRCSC, FACS
Professor, Pediatric Surgery, McMaster University

"This book is BRILLIANT!!!

The addiction families, individuals, field, programs, and research groups are so blessed to have you both introducing to the world how best to provide a REAL living approach to hope and healing and renewal of life. It provides hope and a proven system for those seeking a transformative approach to recovery and healing.

After working for over twenty-five years in the mainstream medical model of mental health and addictions, I knew that we as care providers were missing a key element in a person's journey of recovery and wellbeing.

I began searching for something that could truly help people transform their lives without the use of medications - the brain-first approach - and *Actualized Recovery* did just that!

It was a privilege to work with Dave and Susan where I was introduced to and immersed in their Brain-First, *Actualized Recovery* program. This experience allowed me to witness firsthand lives being positively impacted in a matter of weeks."

- Debbie Wilkes, RSSW, Mental Health & Wellbeing Counsellor, Brain Tech Coach

"An important examination of the primacy of the brain in all that we do, all that we are, and all that we can become. It's refreshing to read a well-reasoned book like *Actualized Recovery* because it discusses vital topics like brain-body dualism and neuroplasticity from a pragmatic and user-friendly point of view that I believe people can benefit from straight out of the box."

- Ted Perkins, Founder &
President of *Recovery Movie Meet-Ups*
Author of *Addicted In Film*
Movies We Love About the Habits We Hate

"For anyone who is struggling with addiction or supporting someone who is, *Actualized Recovery* is a must read!!! Dave and Susan have identified the critical role the brain plays in addiction and how a brain-first approach can support recovery. Actualized Recovery provides an evidence-based, proven, holistic program to support long-lasting change and well-being."

- Noah Gentner, Ph.D., NBC-HWC,
ICF-PCC, CPHWC, HCA-RHC
Program Coordinator - Wellness Coaching Post
Graduate Certificate
Professor, Wellness Coaching/Fitness and Health
Promotion/Kinesiology
Faculty of Health Sciences and Wellness
Humber Institute of Technology & Advanced Learning/
University of Guelph-Humber

"*Actualized Recovery* is a deeply insightful look at how to move your nervous system out of a state of protection and into a state of real growth".

- Russell Kennedy, The Anxiety MD

"*Actualized Recovery* goes beyond traditional recovery methods. The authors skillfully weave together neuroscience, psychology, and spirituality to create a roadmap for true transformation. The book doesn't just talk about recovery; it provides a comprehensive guide to rewiring your brain and building a life of fulfillment. This book is a must-have for anyone on the path to true recovery and transformation."

- Jody Oslund, RN, Recovered Addict,
Internationally-Certified Crisis & Recovery Coach

"I wholeheartedly endorse Dave & Susan Kenney's book, *Actualized Recovery.*

As a Family Physician, it was refreshing to see the unique perspective that I as a clinician, can take on in providing guidance to an individual who is struggling and lost.

No longer looking at their "problem or addiction" in the forefront with band-aid solutions that don't get to the core of their pain. But rather, delving much deeper to the core from a Brain First Approach makes all the difference for ultimate transformation.

I love that a layperson can enter the world of the brain in this book and better understand its dynamic function and how critical of a role it plays in thoughts to action.

So many times, people think that it's inevitable that they will remain in their current state of despair, depression, sickness, anxiety, addiction, etc., without seeing a way out. They think they are destined to be this way. And this is simply Not true.

As Dave and Susan Kenney eloquently write, rediscovering your strengths, passions, and capabilities that you lost somewhere along your life's path".

I couldn't put this book down, it was easy to follow—even the scientific parts—witty, and many relatable stories.

Through *Actualized Recovery,* Dave and Susan Kenney have shown that we truly do have a choice to regain our POWER.

I recommend that you take on the Recovery Blueprint: physiology, psychology, spirit, connections, and lifestyle to create the life you desire. There are limitless possibilities.

I also invite you to join the Emergo Recovery Community. Nothing is more empowering than to be among people who don't judge, accept you on your terms, and bring positive energy. You can also connect with a coach if you feel you need guidance.

Time to live your EXTRAORDINARY LIFE!"

- Esther Malave, M.D.

Internationally-Certified Crisis & Recovery Coach and Host of Achieving a Better U

"The treasures of truth contained in *Actualized Recovery* represent a truly holistic, transformative, and enriching way of escaping the bondage of addiction. Susan and Dave Kenney have put together a thorough and accurate understanding of the role our brain plays in addiction and recovery and made it accessible to all those seeking true and lasting freedom. You will be amazed at what you discover within these pages. It is truly life-changing!

Susan and Dave Kenney have successfully advanced our understanding of addiction recovery through providing a truly comprehensive approach that considers the whole person and how our brain can become our greatest asset in successful recovery. Actualized Recovery is a must-read for anyone looking to better understand addiction and how to escape its tyranny. This book will change countless lives across the world, bringing about illumination and a more holistic and compassionate understanding of human behavior."

- Jason Roop, PhD
Vice President, Research and Development,
Hometown Health System
Professor of Business and Theology,
Campbellsville University
Founder and CEO,
Center for Trait-Based Transformation

Dedication

To our incredible parents, whose distinct and inspiring journeys have deeply ingrained in us the noble pursuit of serving others. With immense pride and endless gratitude, we honor the remarkable impact you've each made, not only in our lives but in the hearts of countless others. Your dedication and love are the pillars upon which we build our own voyages of love, service, and impact.

Contents

Foreword

Before I jump into introducing this mind-blowing book, I have to say, ... "I absolutely LOVE talking about things like this! It lights up my brain!"

I'm not exactly sure what drives me but ever since I was a kid, I've had this insatiable hunger to really understand how everything works, why it works, or even how it might work better, ...and when I think of the brain, and all of the possibilities it holds, the countless programs it runs which guide us....AUTOMATICALLY to every height or depth of life, from health or illness, happiness or pain, wealth or poverty, recovery or catastrophe, or even to enlightenment or debauchery, I'm all ears.

Yes, these are pretty bold statements.

But think of it for a moment. The space between your ears is what determines the life you lead.

I've always loved the expressions,

- "You're not the tape; you're the tape player,"
- "You're not the program; you're the computer,"
- or in today's terms, perhaps, "you're not the app, you're the phone,"

These simply suggest, "I am bigger and have infinite possibilities beyond the song or program my brain is currently playing.

Susan and Dave's compelling research says I can simply put a new program in, and when the computer of my brain runs it, the results I get will be a lot better.

To be clear, they are talking about upgrading our brain's hard drive, not the software. The hard drive is how your brain functions or how it fires. The software is your thoughts, your mindset, or your conscious mind. And how your brain functions (like a computer's hard drive) runs the show. If the hard drive crashes or is compromised, it doesn't matter what software you're running. When we upgrade our hard drive, everything works better, faster, and with less energy or effort.

I subscribe fully and completely to this philosophy.

Not only can you change the tape, the program, and the app, but you can actually upgrade your brain's hard drive or its function (how it works). And that's called neuroplasticity—your brain's ability to re-wire itself.

In 2008, I bought my first iPhone. It was insane. What it could do was beyond anything I had access to before, but compared to my iPhone 13, it's almost laughable. Yes, I have far better apps running on my phone now than I did in 2008, but come on—can I really compare the phone I have today to my first iPhone?

My first-ever iPhone did not have the capacity (the hard drive) to run all the apps and do all the things my new iPhone13 can do. Not even close.

We know if we ate well, slept well, and were constantly of service to others if we immediately cut out thoughts that don't serve us and instead we entertained thoughts that do, we'd lead better, more joyful lives.

Why don't we? Is it because we're lazy, undisciplined, or something else? Well, there is hope. But, although I firmly believe it's something we need, the answer isn't just more discipline.

What if your core thoughts and desires—like a new app on your phone— programmed you to "Do the things you should and don't do the things you shouldn't?"

What you're going to learn is that 'It's not about willpower—it's all about brain power.'

Needless to say, the work of Susan and Dave is beyond cool; it's innovative and will take the recovery world by storm!

How Exactly Is This Possible? How Do We Re-Wire the Brain?

You may be familiar with the phrase: "Thoughts lead to feelings, and feelings lead to actions." Dave and Susan say that's only part of the story. The most important part is being ignored or not understood. We've left out the brain! They say, "Your (potentially broken) brain is generating menacing thoughts, and those thoughts lead to negative feelings, and those feelings lead to negative actions (drinking, drugs, gambling, shopping, anger/rage, isolation, etc)

This is why they're adamant about saying, **"Brain-First,"** and it's the beginning and most important part of their proprietary methodology called "Actualized Recovery®."

Actualized Recovery is a "brain-first" but not "brain only" approach leveraging the latest in neuroscience, physiology, psychology, spirituality, connections, and lifestyle. The results speak for themselves in treating their clients for addiction and trauma and overall increasing their happiness.

Self-destructive behaviors are only a symptom of the problem. These negative choices aren't your fault. As you'll learn from this power-packed book, when a brain is in a state of dysfunction, people tend to find and abuse substances or self-destructive behaviors as a way to seek relief or to self-medicate, regardless of negative outcomes.

Actualized Recovery is about helping clients discover and begin to build a life that matters, one that is rich with meaning and automatically allows them to... "flourish." You gotta love that word, "flourish!" It's all summarized in a single word I'd never heard before, and I had to look it up because it's "Dave's favorite word,"... "Eudaimonia."

Eudaimonia (You-Dah-Monia) is a Greek term coined by Aristotle, meaning "the flourishing life" or "the good life." It's NOT some temporary substance-induced high or an emotional state or even a sense of pleasure, but rather a fulfilled life lived in accordance with a person's deepest values and aspirations – and it's the premise for everything that Actualized Recovery embodies.

It's considered the highest human good, which is desirable for its own sake rather than for the sake of something else. It provides a framework for life-long challenges where improvements are always possible. And it's no surprise those pursuing this recover from addiction, overcome their trauma, and find themselves leading fulfilling and happy lives. No wonder it's Dave's favorite word!

Susan and Dave had saved and re-wired the brains of thousands of clients using their proprietary Actualized Recovery program in their successful residential treatment center. Then, the Covid lockdowns.

They believe and teach that 'Life Happens for Me, Not to Me.'

So, they reflected and realized the Covid shutdown may be an opportunity for something more significant; they thought, "Maybe it's a gift of sorts." And so came the lightbulb and the pivot. "What if?"

Because their background before recovery was education, they saw the opportunity to take their entire Actualized Recovery tested and proven methodology and serve the global masses! And the result is the book that you're about to dive into.

Rob Hannley
Editor in Chief, Recovery Today Magazine

PART 1

NEURO-ARCHITECTURE

Chapter 1

Luctor et Emergo

Latin phrase meaning

I Struggle and I Emerge

The phone rings. It's late. And it's been a long, draining day. But we answer it.

"Hello..."

"I need help. I'm desperate. I don't want to feel like a failure anymore, but I need help."

"I understand, can you explain more?"

"I'm at my wits' end. I don't know what to do. I've tried everything, and nothing has worked. Some things have helped for a short period, but now I feel worse than ever. I feel like giving up. My life seems over."

For over a decade, we got phone calls like this at all hours of the day and night. A crisis doesn't take a holiday.

We've had thousands of calls from mothers, fathers, spouses, life partners, aunts, uncles, grandparents, frantic friends, adult children, and even concerned colleagues. Sometimes it was the person who was struggling. We could hear the pain, despair, and deep worry in their voices. Some were angry and frustrated that it felt like no one was truly listening. Many apologized for their tears while telling us about their paralyzing levels of fear, shame, and hopelessness.

For many of the people who called us, their candle was flickering.

Journey to Recovery

What we've learned on our incredible journey of running a holistic residential recovery and wellness program is that almost every attempt to seek professional help, treatment, or relief is one-dimensional. People are complex beings, multidimensional, and we are interconnected physically, psychologically, and spiritually.

A person struggling with an addiction or Substance Use Disorder (SUD) *(note: we will use either of these phrases interchangeably throughout this book)* is advised to seek help to stop using or abusing the substance. There are very few programs or processes that explore the true WHY behind someone using a substance or the causal self-destructive, catastrophic behavior. Few professionals ask the question, "What is the pain that you're trying to avoid or numb that is driving this need for relief?"

People struggling with various mental health issues are often provided with rushed treatment which, at best, merely manages the symptoms, many times with only a prescription, and they are left with so many unanswered questions. Rarely is the underlying cause addressed.

Even behavioral addictions, sometimes referred to as *soft addictions,* can lead to devastating and life-threatening situations. Yet these are also typically treated as a one-dimensional problem.

It is omnipotent that we unpack some key phrases or definitions as clearly as possible, so we all have the same understanding and framework.

Foundation of Trauma

Every person whose story we heard had a foundation of deep, traumatic events or experiences that had come to the ultimate tipping point. These stories were shared because people trusted us and let us into the darkest corners of their lives.

It was oftentimes gut-wrenching, sometimes heartbreaking to hear their story, yet we remained focused on asking curious questions and listening for key pieces of information to better understand their pain and to offer hope.

Actualized Recovery

The brain-first approach of Actualized Recovery represents a transformative shift in how we address and heal from addiction and self-destructive behaviors. It acknowledges the brain's pivotal role in driving behavior and leverages this powerful insight to realize recovery and the ability to overcome self-destructive habits. By prioritizing the brain's health and function, this methodology addresses the root causes of these challenges and empowers individuals with the tools and knowledge to foster long-lasting change. Integrating neuroscience, mind-body therapies, and holistic lifestyle practices creates a comprehensive pathway toward recovery that is adaptable and evolves with the individual's progress. This approach is more than just a treatment; it's a journey toward a healthier, more harmonious life, where the brain leads the way to a sustained state of wellbeing and thriving. Actualized Recovery is a testament to the resilience and adaptability of the human brain, offering hope and a concrete path forward for those seeking to reclaim control and vibrancy in their lives.

Actualized Recovery offers an innovative approach that brings a deeper, more meaningful understanding to the quest for healing and personal growth as it relates to overcoming addictions or self-destructive behaviors and patterns. Let's break it down into its two core components: *Actualized* and *Recovery.*

Defining *Actualized*

Actualized embodies the journey from potential to reality, a powerful concept that resonates deeply in the context of recovery. It's about converting the seeds of possibility into tangible, impactful results. When we speak of something being actualized, it signifies that it has transcended from mere thought or aspiration into reality. Becoming their reality, or their life.

In the realm of recovery, the essence of actualization takes on a profound meaning. It's not just about the possibility of healing; it's about actualizing that healing into a lived experience. This process is similar to the healing process of a broken bone - it's not just the expectation of mending, but the actual restoration of function and strength. The neat thing is, once the bone has healed, it is often stronger than before the trauma, symbolizing not only a return to the former state but also an evolution into something more resilient.

Actualization in recovery goes beyond physical healing. It's about transforming the suppressed potential for emotional and psychological healing into a reality. This means not just *hoping* to overcome trauma, addiction, or self-destructive patterns, but *manifesting* a state of wellness and stability in their place. It involves actively engaging in practices, therapies, and lifestyle changes that convert the hope of recovery into a genuine state of being.

To actualize recovery is to see beyond the horizon of one's current state and to bring into being a new chapter of life where healing is not just a concept but a living, breathing reality. It's a journey that recognizes and honors the depth of one's challenges, yet also harnesses the incredible power of the human spirit to rebuild, renew, and flourish.

In this way, actualization becomes a pivotal aspect of the recovery process. It's about making the healing process real and experiential, empowering individuals to envision a life beyond their struggles and step into that life with confidence and conviction. Actualized Recovery bridges the potential for wellness and the realization of a life marked by resilience, fulfillment, and profound wellbeing.

Defining *Recovery*

At its essence, *recovery* is about returning to a state of wellness and success, especially after facing setbacks, illnesses, or challenges. It encompasses:

- The act of healing and improvement
- The process of regaining what was lost, whether it's health, stability, or something else of value
- The path to returning to a state of normalcy or success after crisis
- The process or act of getting something back

Recovery isn't just a concept limited to physical ailments like a broken bone or financial difficulties. It also applies to overcoming trauma (physical, mental, chemical, or emotional), addictions or SUDs, and self-destructive habits or behaviors. In this book, we focus on recovery as a holistic process that begins with the brain, understanding that true healing starts by optimizing the engine of your choices – your brain.

Real Recovery in Actualized Recovery

> That's why we call this process Recovery; we recover the YOU that you were meant to be.
>
> \- Russell Brand

Bringing these two concepts together, Actualized Recovery is about making your recovery journey real and sustainable. It's about moving beyond just the aspiration to heal and creating a quantifiable path to live the life you are meant to lead. It's a commitment to transform potential healing into a reality, covering everything from trauma and addictions to self-destructive patterns.

Actualized Recovery is a beacon of hope, a roadmap, and a proven pathway to genuine, lasting recovery. It's about giving you the expertise and knowledge for you to take control of your life, optimizing your brain's health and functionality, and actualizing a future of extraordinary wellbeing. This book is your guide on this transformative journey, giving you hope and helping you not just dream of recovery but to make it a lived actualized reality.

Brain-First Approach

The *brain-first* approach of Actualized Recovery has helped people overcome trauma, grief, obsessive-compulsive disorder (OCD), dependency, addictions or SUDs, mental health challenges, self-destructive patterns, drifting, negative choices, and many other life-limiting behaviors. You'll learn much more about the brain-first approach in Chapter 5.

Defining Trauma

Trauma can manifest and present in distinctive ways, including physically, mentally, chemically, and/or emotionally.

Physical trauma refers to any physical injury or harm to the body caused by an external force or event, such as accidents, falls, injury, disrupted homeostasis, surgeries, disease, inflammation, malnutrition, chronic pain, or physical assault. Physical trauma can lead to a range of physical symptoms, such as pain, swelling, bruising, and impaired or limited mobility.

Mental trauma refers to the psychological impact of experiencing or witnessing a distressing event, such as a natural disaster, war, violent crime, or an event perceived as threatening. Mental trauma can result in symptoms such as anxiety, depression, post-traumatic stress disorder (PTSD), addiction, and many other mental health conditions.

Chemical trauma can occur when the person has contracted a virus or bacterial infection, has had a fever, experiences adrenaline surges, blood sugar dysregulation; when the body has accumulated toxins, been exposed to poisons, some medications, substances, or has heavy metal deposits that are causing physiological or emotional symptoms.

Emotional trauma refers to the psychological distress of experiencing or witnessing an event that causes emotional duress, such as abuse, feeling unsafe, tragedy, drama, shock, emotional dysregulation, neglect, the loss of a loved one, financial ruin, or security. Emotional trauma can lead to symptoms such as feelings of shame, guilt, anger, isolation, confusion, grief, sadness, and difficulty forming or maintaining relationships.

Traumatic events, whether real or perceived, can adversely impact the brain and central nervous system, causing a cascade of unwanted negative issues.

Addictions/Substance Use Disorder

We are going to explore this in much more detail in a future chapter, but for now, here is a snapshot:

Addiction is a complex and chronic condition characterized by compulsive behavior despite negative consequences and an inability to avoid, control, or limit the use of a substance or behavior. Addiction can involve the use of substances like drugs or alcohol, as well as behaviors such as gambling, gaming, drama, scrolling, or shopping.

Addiction can have significant negative impacts on an individual's physical, emotional, and social wellbeing. It can lead to degenerative health problems, financial difficulties, legal issues or arrests, relationship problems, the need to withdraw and isolate, suicide ideation, premature death, and so many more unfavorable consequences.

> Addiction can be defined as the inability to control or manage behavior or choice.

It is worth noting that compulsive or impulsive behaviors are a commonality regardless of the addiction.

Addiction can be characterized by a person's *inability to control or manage behavior or choice*. This can manifest in the use or abuse of substances like alcohol, tobacco, drugs, or food or can include engaging in behaviors such as shopping, pornography, self-harm, gambling, etc. Losing the ability to regulate or moderate behavior (choices), particularly when facing harmful consequences, is the essence of addiction.

This straightforward explanation does not delve into the underlying reasons or root causes of addiction. Still, it captures the behavioral pattern where individuals find themselves trapped in a cycle of addiction, often to the detriment of their wellbeing.

The individual may gain or feel a sense of relief from consuming a substance or repeating a behavior, but any sense of relief is short-term, at best. Oftentimes, the person can not imagine their life without this form of consumption and as a result, they will resist intervention to continue having this short-lived reprieve of pain or discomfort, often at the sacrifice of things they value to keep this form of relief in their lives, despite adverse outcomes.

Self-Destructive Patterns, Habits, or Choices

Self-destructive habits are behaviors that can harm an individual's physical, psychological, spiritual, or social wellbeing. These behaviors may be intentional or unintentional, adversely impacting a person's life and relationships.

Some examples may include failure to launch, self-harm or threatening self-harm, eating disorders, lying, anger/rage, isolation, drifting, procrastination, incessant tardiness, disregard for others, poor personal hygiene, dangerous driving habits, risky behaviors, chaos, poor nutrition choices, stealing/theft or other illegal activities, constant drama, infidelity, and more.

Why does someone choose negative behaviors despite a desire to change? One answer could be that they truly don't want to change. Another explanation, which we will explore in greater detail and is more likely, is that the brain has been hardwired through repeated reinforcing actions. These resulting dominant brain patterns then become automatic, like riding a bike. In short, how the brain functions drives conduct that overrides willpower.

The Tip of the Iceberg

We have developed an 'Iceberg' metaphor to better understand this interconnected approach.

Since 2011, thousands of people have contacted us, asking if we can help solve their problem or crisis.

What we've come to realize is that problems - like addictions or self-destructive patterns/habits - are merely the tip of the iceberg. Roughly ninety percent of an iceberg is beneath the waterline, leaving only ten percent exposed at the top. Therefore, the problems that we tend to focus on are only on the tip, also known as *surface issues*.

Most efforts to help people are focused on the problem. 12-step programs, for example, are focused solely on the symptoms or problem, i.e. alcohol, drugs, gambling, etc. It is important to note that these are only surface issues.

As shown in the illustration, when the storm (the addictions, trauma, and self-destructive habits) is raging, it's only bashing into the tip of the iceberg.

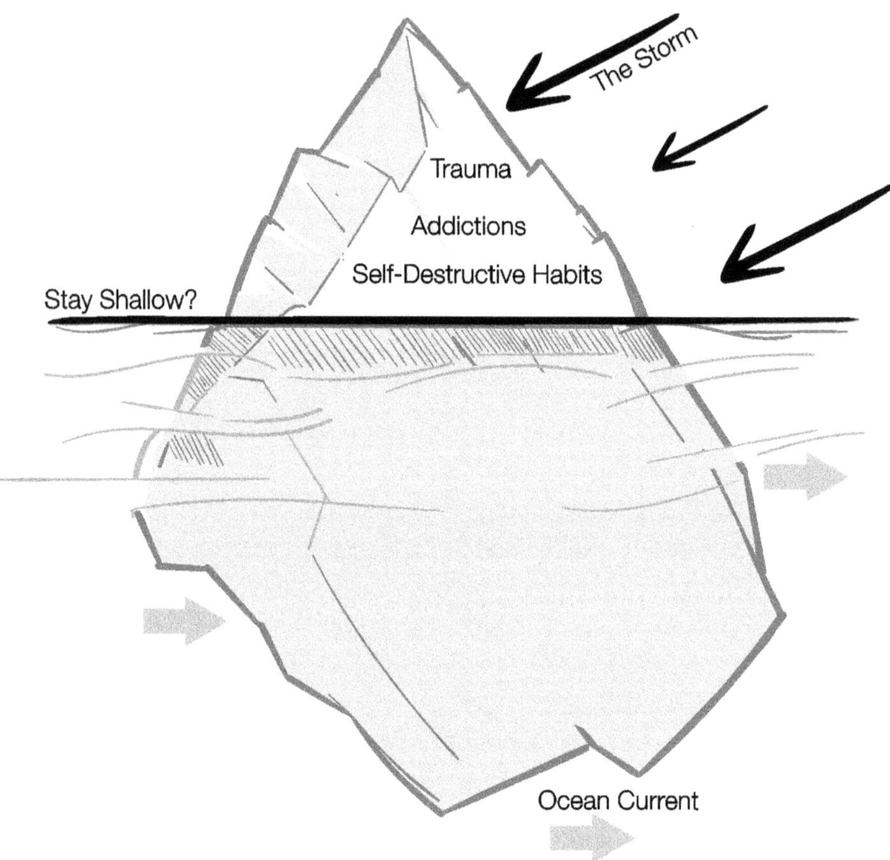

The wind, waves, or storms crashing into the tip of an iceberg do not matter. They are simply not going to move an iceberg. The direction or movement of an iceberg depends on the currents far below the surface.

The solutions that are typically recommended either don't last or don't address the deeper root cause because they are only a short-term band-aid solution that reacts to and focuses on the current crisis. Therefore, these solutions represent a shallow approach.

Let's Go Deeper

The true *power* of an iceberg resides beneath the surface. Do you want to focus on surface issues and stay shallow, or do you want to go deeper for lasting solutions?

The wind and storm can be raging above the surface, yet immediately below the waterline, the ocean current controls the direction of the iceberg. Here, at the deeper level—below the waterline—you can implement real change.

After working with thousands of people in crisis, we have recognized three critical outcome areas we define as the goals of Actualized Recovery. These three outcomes are the summary of what people genuinely want. The three outcomes of Actualized Recovery drive real change, growth, healing, and transformation. When you focus on a problem, you get more problems.

When clients first step into our program, we often ask them a simple yet profound question: "If we had a magic wand and we could fix or change one thing in your life right now, what is that one thing?" The overwhelming response? *"I just want to be happy."*

Regardless of what debilitating challenge they were struggling with, whether that was alcohol, drugs, suicide ideation, legal or court problems, self-harming, gambling, rage, eating disorders, and more, their response was consistent. Using nearly identical words time and time again they would say *"I just want to be happy."*

When given one wish, no one said they wanted to get rid of depression, anxiety, shame, guilt, fear, or addiction. People intuitively know that the deeper solution is not about stopping or changing a behavior; it is a deep desire to realize their happiness. Quite frankly, why change any behavior if you do not reach a greater point of happiness or wellbeing?

One of the strengths of this approach is focusing on what people want, not what they don't want.

This led us to look deeper and uncover core outcomes, allowing people to rise above and realize greater meaning and happiness. And this is how we create an inspirational comeback story.

Actualized Recovery – Core Outcomes

When we go deeper, the three core outcomes came about because of our work and our incredible teams of recovery coaches, emotional and energy therapists, personal trainers, medical professionals, social workers, chefs, and many others over the years, discovering with people what they truly wanted their lives to be and how that was different from the way they had been living.

We noticed an overlap in what everyone desired and what they deeply yearned for in their life and for their future.

The three core outcomes are:

1) Epic Wellbeing
2) Heroic Autonomy
3) Vibrant Longevity

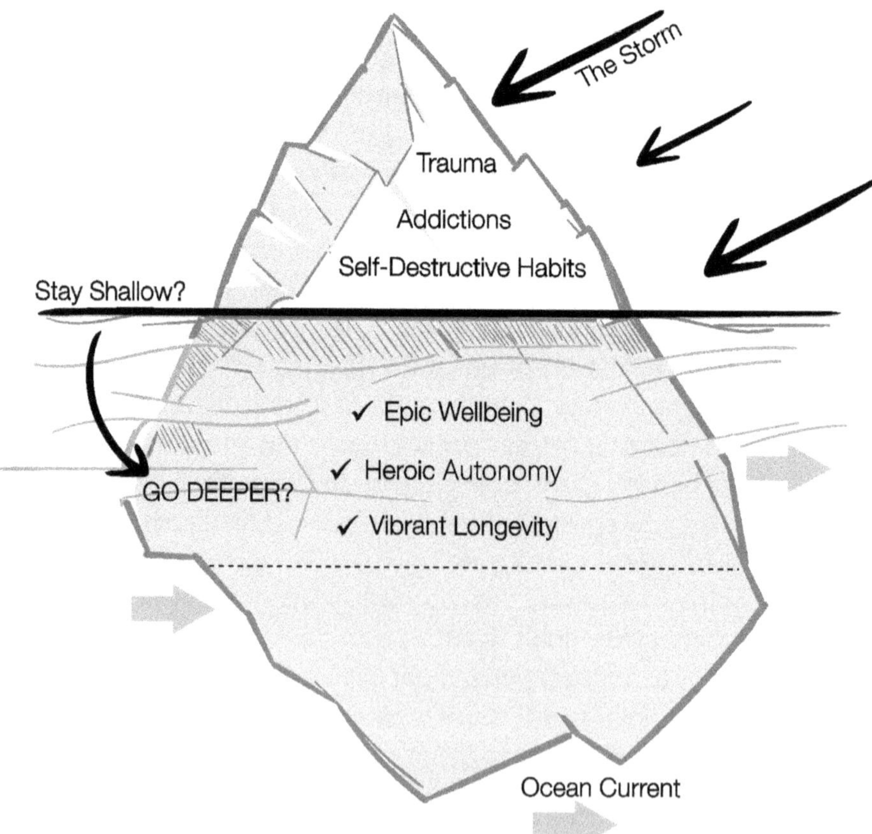

Epic Wellbeing

Firstly, our clients wanted to feel healthy and well. They wanted to have meaningful relationships with family and friends. They wanted to enjoy prosperity and have enough to take care of themselves and those they loved. They wanted to thrive in a career that excited them and made them feel proud of their accomplishments. They wanted to have adventures, laugh, play, and celebrate life.

It's about more than just stopping a harmful habit; it's about cultivating a life where you feel genuinely good, both inside and out. When you focus on your overall wellbeing, you're not just addressing the physical aspect of addiction, but also nurturing your mental and emotional health. This holistic approach provides a solid foundation for lasting recovery. It helps build resilience against triggers and stresses, improves self-esteem, and fosters a positive mindset. Striving toward epic wellbeing means embracing a life where you're not just free from addiction, but where you thrive, enjoying a fulfilling and balanced life.

Heroic Autonomy

Secondly, it was important for everyone to live a life whereby they could make their own decisions and choices, to be free of dependence on substances, cigarettes, junk food, drama, governments, and other people's resources, and to live an independent and self-sustaining life. They wanted freedom of personal choice and not to be told what to do – they wanted to stop being a victim and create their own destiny. They wanted to learn the skills of resilience to ride life's ups and downs.

Students are not taught how to live or achieve this in school; most families struggle to teach and live this concept. What we discovered was almost all families played a key role in creating a victim with greater dependency.

Embracing autonomy means empowering oneself to make choices that align with personal values and long-term wellness.

It represents taking personal control and making independent decisions, which is crucial for breaking free from the cycles of dependency. This can be scary because with greater independence comes greater responsibility. However, this is also where freedom lies—freedom from substances, freedom from self-destructive choices, freedom from negative relationships—to live your life on your terms.

Vibrant Longevity

Thirdly, our clients wanted to create a life that mattered to them and others and at the end of their time on earth, know that they had made a difference to those they cared about and created something greater that outlived them. They wanted to develop moral character and be trusted – to live a life true to themselves and their values. It was important to many that they support the causes that were meaningful to them by having an abundance of resources to be able to share. They wanted to have faith and feel connected to something beyond the physical – to live fulfilling their destiny. Some wanted to achieve status to obtain recognition. They wanted to be fearless.

Longevity in overcoming addiction is pivotal for thriving in life. It's not just short-term wins or a temporary solution. Focusing on longevity is building a sustainable lifestyle that supports continuous growth and wellbeing. Consider if you want to become more physically fit. You may choose to change your diet and incorporate exercise and mindfulness practices; the key is consistent long-term action. Longevity is achieved by incorporating these practices into your lifestyle and optimizing how you think, look, and feel. It's not a flash-in-the-plan solution.

Actualized Recovery creates the opportunity for you to embrace your growth and embody your new lifestyle so you can thrive. Now that's vibrant longevity!

Whatever crisis or hardship an individual faces, we can lead, coach, and inspire them to embrace and customize these three outcomes. Focusing on what you want is when miracles can happen.

Take a minute or two to reflect on the following question.

Clear your mind. Allow yourself to release any stories, excuses, limiting beliefs, and rationalizations. Let your thoughts go and dream big for a few minutes. Focus on what you *want*, not what you *don't want*.

Coaching Tip:

Take three deep slow breathes (slowly in....hold....slowly out). Do this three times. Now ask yourself this...
How would my life be impacted if I were to fully embrace and live each day with

- Epic Wellbeing,
- Heroic Autonomy,
- and Vibrant Longevity?

How do you imagine your life would change?

What would this really mean for you and your family? Be specific.

Write your answers in a journal or somewhere important for you. Without judgment, suspend any limiting beliefs (I can't do that), dream a little. Now write your thoughts, your emotions, and your vision.

When you work below the distracting tip of the iceberg at a deeper level, you are no longer living a reactive life. You are seizing your power, launching full speed ahead on your hero's journey.

The Base of the Iceberg

As incredible as these three outcomes are, there is an even deeper level. While Epic Wellbeing, Heroic Autonomy, and Vibrant

Longevity are extremely important, it isn't only about these. When you have these, you unlock something even more incredible.

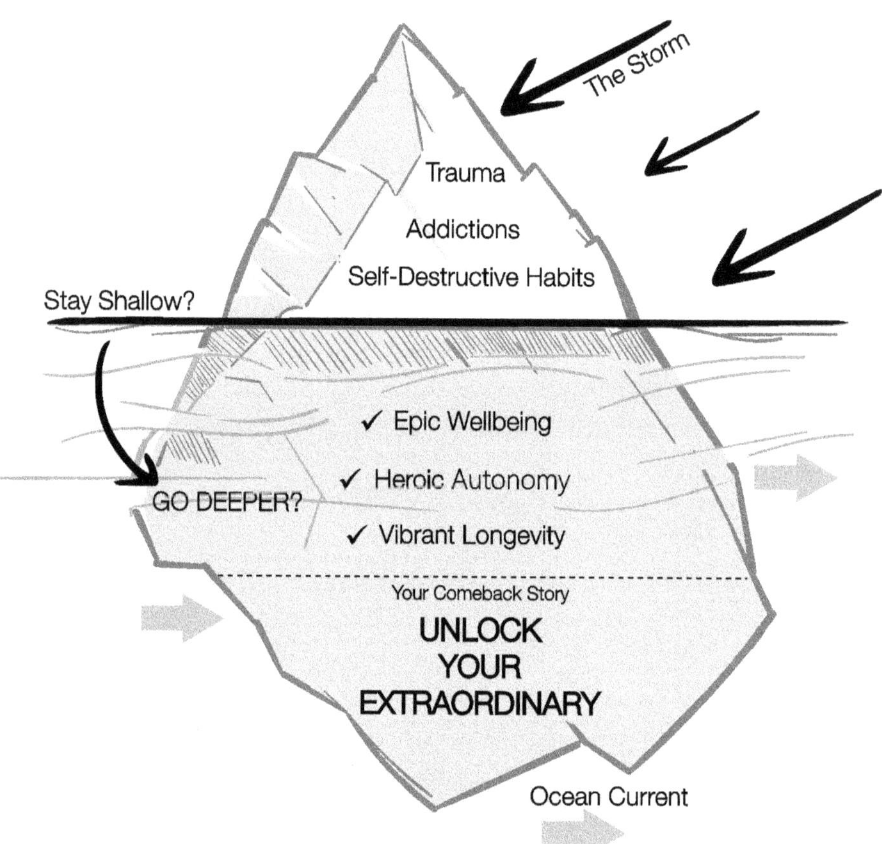

Here is what we believe: The awe-inspiring transformations we've witnessed again and again are possible for you and for everyone.

You deserve the opportunity to ***Unlock Your Extraordinary***!

Isn't that what you really want? Isn't that what you truly deserve?

This is your comeback story!

In life, it is not about where you are, it is about your choice to move forward... or not. We call this free will, or free won't. So many of the greatest stories and Hollywood movies are about overcoming adversity and challenge – it's the comeback story. The classic holiday movie *A Christmas Carol* illustrates Ebenezer Scrooge's comeback. Of course, there is *Rocky*, an inspirational comeback movie. But it's not just in the movies - the best comebacks happen in real everyday life.

In 1980, a team of struggling university underdog athletes took on the USSR (Russian) hockey team. At that time, the USSR hockey team was unbeatable and one of the most powerful hockey teams in the history of the game. Yet this team of university athletes overcame many challenges and shockingly beat Team USSR to go on and win the gold medal at the Lake Placid Olympics. This story took the nation by storm.

Everyone loves a comeback story! It is one of the things that makes humanity great, it unites us. Against all odds, we triumph and inspire others to do the same. This is the human experience.

When you courageously look forward and leave what's behind you in the rear-view mirror, you're no longer stuck and paralyzed in your past problems. You are no longer focusing on the tip of the iceberg. You can achieve heroic possibilities when you go deeper, focusing your efforts on what you want.

Now, we are going to reveal how you can rise above your painful struggles and how you can *Unlock Your Extraordinary.*

Chapter 2

The Untold Truth

Change Your Brain, Change Your Life.

- Daniel Amen, MD

Think back and recall a trip. A trip where you were brimming with excitement and anticipation. One where you had to fly. Maybe it was to the Caribbean for a glorious beach vacation at a 5-star resort. Maybe it was a trip to Paris or the rolling green hills of Ireland. Maybe it was a Thanksgiving trip to visit family and loved ones.

The morning of your trip goes off without a hitch. Traffic is light. You arrive with plenty of time. You check in, and surprisingly, you are offered a free upgrade to the front of the plane. You stroll through security with ease. You stop to buy a drink and snack for the plane. Now you're off to find your departure gate.

You have a few extra minutes, so you wander over to the terminal windows beside your gate to gaze at your aircraft.

But wait....what is that?

Parked at the gate you see a plane, your plane, and it's an old-school Douglas DC-3, made in 1935.

It's been well maintained, but nothing has been updated. No aerospace or technology upgrades have been incorporated. It's all original, has a maximum capacity of 21 passengers, and has two propeller engines. And yes, it's your plane.

How do you feel?

What do you do?

Imagine having heart surgery using medical practices, imaging, and technology from 1935.

How about using a telephone from 1935?

The list goes on. We can use so many colorful metaphors to illustrate that staying current with technology, science, medicine, education, communication, construction, travel, and more is both critical and something we all greatly value.

Air travel has enhanced the proven fundamental concepts of flight, making it safer, faster, more enjoyable, and more affordable.

It seems wise that we would all want the benefits of today's advances in science, medicine, technology, psychology, nutrition, mindfulness, lifestyle medicine, and more to help us overcome any personal adversity or struggle, including recovering from the shackles of addiction so that we may live our best life, being our best self.

History of Alcoholics Anonymous

Alcoholics Anonymous (AA) is a global organization that provides support to individuals who struggle with alcohol addiction. Founded in 1935 by Bill Wilson (Bill W.) and Dr. Bob Smith, AA started as a small group of individuals who sought to recover from alcoholism through mutual support.

The origins of AA can be traced back to the personal experiences of Bill Wilson, who had struggled with alcohol addiction for many years. In 1934, Wilson had a spiritual awakening that he believed freed him from the grip of alcoholism. He sought out other alcoholics to help them achieve sobriety using his newfound approach. He found little success.

In May 1935, Wilson met Dr. Bob Smith, a surgeon who also suffered from alcoholism. The two men shared their experiences and found that they had a lot in common. They agreed to work together to help other alcoholics achieve sobriety.

The first meeting of Alcoholics Anonymous took place on June 10, 1935, in Akron, Ohio. The 12-step program was initially based on the Oxford Group, a Christian spiritual movement that emphasized the principles of moral inventory, confession, restitution, and guidance. By incorporating these principles, the AA founders laid out a path for personal transformation and moral living as the framework for their program.

In 1939, Wilson and Smith published the book *Alcoholics Anonymous*. This book details their approach to recovery and includes the 12-step program that has become synonymous with AA. The 12 steps are a set of principles that guide individuals through a process, beginning with admitting powerlessness over alcohol, seeking help from a higher power, and ending with a commitment to help others who suffer from addiction.

As word of AA spread, the organization grew rapidly. By 1941, there were over 100 AA groups in the United States. The first international group was established in Toronto, Canada, and had its first meeting on January 13, 1943. Today, there are over two million members of AA worldwide, and the organization has become an iconic part of the recovery community.

Bill W. did get sober and never drank again. But even though Bill wasn't drinking, he was still struggling in life. Bill suffered from the *black dog of depression* and anxiety. One can ask which one was first? Did his deep depression drive the drinking, or was alcohol the precursor to his depression? This has never been clearly established. What is known is that Bill W. remained sober for years while still suffering from paralyzing bouts of depression and anxiety.

Around 1945, he stepped away from AA and appointed a board of directors to oversee the organization. It was an international board comprised primarily of doctors.

Introducing Vitamin Therapy - Niacin (Vitamin B3)

In 1960, Bill W. attended a conference in New York City as he continued on his journey of seeking relief. He met two esteemed psychiatrists, Dr. Abram Hoffer from Weyburn, Saskatchewan, and Dr. Humphry Osmond. They were presenting new findings, specifically about vitamin B3 (also known as niacin) and how it was shown to reverse symptoms of people with schizophrenia and alcohol addiction. They presented a theory called mega-dosing and taught that when the brain is deficient in specific vitamins and minerals, it can impair brain function, hamper wellbeing, and drive a chronic state of illness.

Bill W. began taking mega dosages of niacin daily. Within fourteen days, he reported that his anxiety and depression were gone. His wife corroborated this. Ponder this for a moment... in a mere fourteen days, Bill W. self-reported that his lifelong battle with depression and anxiety was no more.

Bill W. was overjoyed. However, he knew he had a test group of one, which in science is empty and meaningless. He chose to go back to the hospitals where people were struggling with extreme alcohol addiction. He proceeded to introduce vitamin B3 therapy to a group of volunteers. He ended up working with approximately 65 individuals, all struggling with alcohol addiction. They began taking large doses of vitamin B3.

Within 30 days, about one-third of that group was depression-free, symptom-free, and felt better than ever, and stopped drinking alcohol. Another one-third of the group took about 90 days to report that they were feeling amazing; their depression had lifted, and they had no cravings to drink alcohol. The final one-third of the group still reported that they had depression, even though they weren't drinking any longer.

That means that two-thirds—approximately a 66% efficacy rate—experienced the alleviation of both depression symptoms and cravings simply from using vitamin B3 – all in 90 days or less!

Bill W. was elated; he then took his findings to the international board of AA, a group he had hand-picked to oversee AA and most of whom he considered friends. With great enthusiasm, he presented these astonishing outcomes to the board. The response was to criticize him and turn him away, stating that because he had no professional medical designation, he didn't have the credibility to extoll the virtues of vitamin therapy.

Bill W. worked diligently for the next 11 years to spread the word about the efficacy of niacin therapy, but sadly, he never gained any traction. He died in 1971 from pneumonia. His wife, Lois Wilson, documented and shared Bill's findings, confirming that he remained depression-free, anxiety-free, and alcohol-free for the remainder of his life after vitamin therapy and the positive effects it had on his brain and mood.

AUTHORS' NOTE – IMPORTANT

The above story is used to illustrate what Bill Wilson chose to do and the events that led up to and after his vitamin therapy.

We, the authors of this book, are not recommending vitamin B3 dosing or mega-dosing. Any such decisions must be made under the direct consultation of a doctor or licensed medical practitioner (as determined by your state or province).

Under the direction of licensed medical practitioners, our clients have reported, and we have witnessed, positive physical and psychological benefits with vitamin therapy (also called orthomolecular therapy) as determined and administered by a qualified and fully licensed practitioner.

We do not make medical recommendations, nor do we provide any medical advice whatsoever. We strongly urge you to consult with your doctor or licensed health care provider for any medical advice.

AA is based on spiritual principles and fellowship, with its roots in the Oxford Group (a spiritually based group).

AA and all 12-step programs globally have endeavored to help millions of people, and if a 12-step approach has served you or a loved one, we applaud that.

The 12-steps were created in the absence of the evolving and most recent scientific findings in the field of addiction and recovery research. There was no evidence of the brain and behavioral connection in 1935. The scientific world did not commonly accept neuroplasticity (the brain's ability to change by rewiring itself) until the late 1990s. Mr. Wilson and Dr. Smith did their best to create a model to help those in pain struggling with alcohol addiction (then called *alcoholism*).

The 12-step programs lack the benefit of today's scientific evidence. In almost 90 years since the creation of the AA 12-step model, Alcoholics Anonymous has not adapted, changed, or modified this model to reflect science (specifically addiction science), neuroscience, psychology, positive psychology, or other evidence-based behavioral disciplines.

There is no other medical illness, disease, disorder, or even behavioral dysfunction whose treatment or care plan has remained entrenched with what we believed almost a century ago.

Is there value in a spiritual foundation and faith? Absolutely yes! In fact, one of the five principles of Actualized Recovery is Spirit, which some consider to be faith. Yet, no reasonable person would pursue a higher power solely as a means of dealing with an illness, disease, disorder, or even a behavioral problem. To do so would be a tunnel vision approach that disregards the remarkable evolution of science, specifically neuroscience.

For instance, most people would not turn to fellowship and a higher power as their sole means of dealing with diabetes, heart disease, lung illness, etc. This may seem an irresponsible, risky, and irrational approach to health, wellbeing, and longevity.

Another strength of AA is its emphasis on fellowship. The numerous benefits of fellowship and meaningful connections are crucial in overcoming significant challenges, such as alcohol or other addictions.

As inherently social beings, we flourish with strong personal connections. This concept is powerfully examined in Johann Hari's book, *Lost Connections: Why You're Depressed and How to Find Hope*. Hari delves into how connections bolster mental wellbeing, and how their absence can have a detrimental, cascading effect on mental health. The study of *happiness* often highlights deep, meaningful relationships as a critical component, as they provide emotional support and a sense of belonging and enrich people's lives. These relationships contribute significantly to our overall wellbeing and happiness, fulfilling essential psychological needs for connection and validation. In our work, we firmly believe in the significance of deep, meaningful relationships and connections as a foundational principle for lasting recovery.

Leveraging Modern Evolved Science

Leveraging science for your physical, emotional, mental, or behavioral wellbeing releases you from shame. Even lifestyle-driven chronic diseases (heart disease, cancer, Type 2 diabetes, etc.) are not met with shame. Instead, they are met with compassion and empathy.

Addictions, both *soft* and *hard*, are branded in fault. They carry a social stigma of harsh judgment for the person and their character, or lack thereof. Some still believe this is a moral failing or a lack of willpower. This condemnation comes from not truly understanding the root cause of addiction and a belief that the addictive pattern or behavior is within complete control of the individual. This conclusion brings with it crushing shame, which only exacerbates the problem.

Science teaches us that the roots of addiction are complex. What has been determined is that a dysfunctional or asymmetric brain sets the stage for many behaviors that are not aligned with the values and morals of the person.

When you attend an AA (or 12-step) meeting, you must introduce and label yourself by defining your infirmity: "Hi, my name is ______ and I'm an alcoholic." Many of you reading this book may remember saying that for the first time. Even if you didn't fully agree with it, you had little choice due to peer pressure and the AA meeting culture. For many, saying these words can feel like you're a brutal failure, wrapped in personal weakness, and feel a punishing and paralyzing cloud of shame.

There is no other physical, mental, or emotional issue where it is the custom to introduce and label yourself as being powerless over your life—in essence, you are a victim without choice. If you go five years or fifty-five years without drinking and you're thriving in all aspects of your life, AA still requires you to label yourself and say that you are powerless, despite evidence to the contrary.

The Sober Truth

Dr. Lance Dodes, a psychologist and psychoanalyst, spent over 35 years in the field of addiction treatment. He has served as the Director of the Substance Abuse Treatment Unit of Harvard's McLean Hospital and taught extensively at Harvard Medical School. In 2014, Dr. Dodes and his son Zachary Dodes co-authored the book *The Sober Truth: Debunking The Bad Science Behind the 12-Step Programs and The Rehab Industry.*

They present addiction as having been treated as a moral failing rather than a medical condition. This approach has led to the harmful stigmatization of addicts and the belief that the addict is responsible for their addiction. In their heavily researched book, the authors demonstrate that this attitude of blame and shame has made it difficult to treat addiction effectively.

Dodes points out that AA's approach is based on spiritual principles and a necessary belief in a higher power. He shares that this approach cannot be effective for everyone. He also digs into the claim that AA's high success rate is based on self-reported data from members and, therefore, does not hold a high level of scientific scrutiny.

Dodes shares several studies that have shown mixed results in the effectiveness of AA. One study he cites found that only about

5% of those who attended AA meetings for the first time were still attending after one year. They go on to suggest that AA has many limitations as an addiction treatment method and that there is a need for more effective and individualized approaches to addiction treatment and the power of adopting evidenced-based approaches.

Let's Get Some Clarity: the Definition of Addiction

What is *addiction*? How is it defined? Unfortunately, there is no one answer or a single definition. Different professional groups reference an addiction by a different name or label. Psychiatrists have renamed addictions *substance use disorders* (SUD). They further sub-categorize different SUDs. Other professional groups call it *substance abuse*. Some groups have identified these issues as *soft addictions* or *hard addictions*. (The purpose of this book is not to debate the names or labels.)

Doctors can accurately define and test for many illnesses, such as chronic kidney disease, heart disease, cancers, diabetes, etc. Having a standard definition provides clarity for people to seek the best treatment for their specific condition or symptoms.

The National Institute on Drug Abuse (NIDA) uses the following definition:

> *Addiction is defined as a chronic, relapsing disorder characterized by compulsive drug seeking and use despite adverse consequences. It is considered a brain disorder, because it involves functional changes to brain circuits involved in reward, stress, and self-control. Those changes may last a long time after a person has stopped taking drugs.*
>
> *Addiction is a lot like other diseases, such as heart disease. Both disrupt the normal, healthy functioning of an organ in the body, both have serious harmful effects, and both are, in many cases, preventable and treatable. If left untreated, they can last a lifetime and may lead to death.*

NIDA clearly defines addiction as a "brain disorder." They draw the parallel that it is similar to diseases like heart disease or other organ-type disease states.

The American Society of Addiction Medicine (ASAM) is North America's largest professional association of medical and addiction clinicians. In September 2019, the ASAM Board of Directors issued a new definition for addiction:

> *Addiction is a treatable, chronic medical disease involving complex interactions among brain circuits, genetics, the environment, and an individual's life experiences. People with addiction use substances or engage in behaviors that become compulsive and often continue despite harmful consequences. Prevention efforts and treatment approaches for addiction are generally as successful as those for other chronic diseases.*
>
> (Source: https://www.asam.org/quality-care/definition-of-addiction)

ASAM identifies addiction as a "chronic medical disease", and they relate their definition to the brain and how the brain fires.

Of interest, the American Medical Association (AMA)—the governing body for all doctors in the US— first classified alcoholism as a disease state in 1956, only to include addiction as a disease state in 1987. It was ASAM who agreed with and joined the AMA defining addiction as a chronic brain disorder, not a behavior problem, nor the result of simply making poor or negative choices.

The National Association for Alcoholism and Drug Abuse Counselors (NAADAC) defines addiction as:

> *A primary, chronic disease of brain reward, motivation, memory, and related circuitry. Addiction is characterized by the inability to consistently abstain from a substance or behavior, despite significant harm to oneself or others. It is often accompanied by cravings, physical dependence, and tolerance, and can lead to negative consequences in various*

areas of an individual's life, such as social, occupational, and health related domains. Addiction is considered a complex and multifaceted disorder that requires comprehensive and individualized treatment to address the unique needs of each person.

Here, NAADAC states addiction is related to brain reward challenges and labels addiction as a "disorder."

The Big Miss

When we consider and contrast the definitions of addiction from these four very legitimate professional bodies with the 12-step model, something does not align, and it is significant; the puzzle pieces just don't fit.

As stated earlier, we acknowledge that Bill W. and his colleagues did their very best in the 1930s to create a program to help themselves and others overcome alcohol addiction. They did not benefit from today's evidence-based approaches and imagery that is revolutionizing the understanding of the human brain and human behavior. Today's neuro-imaging is fascinating and continues to evolve, allowing us to *see* how a brain works.

The evidence is overwhelming; the brain is directly related to addictions (SUD), and thus, the brain must be a central part of any successful recovery modality.

It seems wise and logical to embrace the best of the past with the best evidenced-based findings in understanding addictions (SUD). The goal is to give people hope and a brighter future with integrated, personalized recovery models so they can create their inspirational comeback story and rise above.

A New Understanding of Addiction

Addiction is a *disease*. More recently, new descriptors have emerged, including *disorder*. You can get into a passionate debate as to which term is more accurate.

However, without a single legitimate medical or professional definition that is widely accepted, we are obliged to determine a prevalent thread. Whether you believe it's a disease or a disorder, every professional group worldwide relates addiction to one thing. That one commonality is the brain.

Addiction is not driven by:

- The liver
- The lungs
- The heart
- Genetics
- Or a character defect

Addiction is Not About Willpower or a Higher Power. It's All About Brain Power.

Whether it is a disease, a disorder, or a circuit issue, every legitimate professional organization will agree that addictions are either related to or driven by the brain.

The disciplines of psychology, psychiatry, and neuroscience all agree that the brain drives behavior (more about this in Chapter 4). All these professional fields validate that human behavior *is* driven by the brain, where behavior is defined by an action or response.

Examples of choices defined by action or response:

- What do I choose to do with my life?
- Where do I choose to spend my resources?
- What relationships do I want in my life?
- What adventures do I choose?
- When do I decide to sleep or start my day?
- Do I make my bed?

- Do I choose to go running or swimming, or do I choose to smoke, eat sweets, and watch hours of TV?

These choices define your behavior, and the ability to choose originates from your brain.

Understanding that the brain drives behavior is a critical foundation to begin the conversation because it will likely change how addiction is perceived, therefore creating new opportunities for the world of recovery.

Suppose someone has a brain issue or a brain-driven challenge. In that case, it becomes imperative that we focus our recovery efforts on this specific organ to optimize its level of performance.

The Brain and Trauma

What if using a substance or acting out with a negative behavior is simply about getting relief from pain or trauma? Trauma impacts how the brain processes. Depending on the trauma, it can negatively impact your physical, emotional, or mental wellbeing.

From a brain point of view, trauma can cause the neurological circuitry to become stuck in negative patterns. Whether it's physical, chemical, mental, or emotional trauma, it affects the brain the same way. Trauma is closely linked to stress. It may take one stressful or traumatic event to negatively influence the brain, i.e., a car accident, or it may take multiple stressful events over many years, i.e., emotional or physical abuse.

It's now evident using brain imaging or mapping technology that when brain function is in an asymmetric state, meaning its function becomes unbalanced, this physiological change alters how a person responds, thinks, feels, and acts, just as a heart that is not functioning well impairs the wellbeing of the person and limits what they can achieve to varying degrees.

Your brain's priority, consider it Job #1, is to keep you alive. Your brain is not concerned about whether you feel happy or content or that you remember a new route home from work. Its sole priority is to keep you alive. To stay in balance or harmony, your central nervous system (CNS) has two essential, yet opposite, functions.

Your Brain is the Most Advanced Hard Drive Ever

The CNS is the control center for your body. It's made up of your brain and spinal cord. Think of your brain as your hard drive, and understand that it runs everything you feel, think, and do. Your brain's software is different. The software is the programs and experiences you have which are downloaded into your hard drive (your brain).

If your computer gets hacked and becomes infected with a virus, none of the software will work properly. Your computer will be sluggish, do things it's not supposed to do, and possibly stop functioning altogether. The only way to resolve this is to reset and fix your computer's hard drive. When you restore the hard drive it will work faster, handle more tasks simultaneously, and do so with less energy and effort. That's the benefit of having a kick-ass hard drive.

Your brain is the CEO, making decisions and sending out instructions in a nanosecond (faster than you blink). Your spinal cord is like a super-fast highway, carrying messages between the brain and the rest of your body. Together, they control everything you do, from thinking and feeling to moving and breathing. It's your body's master command system.

Your nervous system has two parts - the sympathetic nervous system (SNS) and the parasympathetic nervous system (PNS). While these two systems complement each other, they react and respond in very different ways.

Your Brain's Gas Pedal – The Fight or Flight Response

The SNS is in charge of regulating the body's "fight or flight" response to stress, danger, or excitement. Think of the SNS as the gas pedal for the nervous system. When activated, it prepares the body to react by increasing heart rate, constricting blood vessels, dilating air passages, and releasing adrenaline and other stress hormones. It is a crucial component of the autonomic nervous system that enables the body to respond to stress and danger. When activated, it alerts the body and sends the message that it's *Go Time*!. While its activation is necessary for survival, chronic activation (without downtime) can have detrimental health consequences. Think of the sympathetic response as a Formula 1 race car – it allows you to go fast, be laser-focused, and be highly alert. Even though the race car is an incredible vehicle, it still needs to go to the pit for service to maintain the pace.

Unfortunately, people stuck in this state, with the gas pedal mashed to the floor all the time, will seek relief at almost any cost.

Your Brain's Brake – The Freeze Response

The PNS is the other primary division of the autonomic nervous system and works in opposition to the SNS. While the SNS prepares the body for action, the PNS helps it relax and conserve energy. It is sometimes referred to as the *rest and digest* system.

You can think of the PNS as the brain's brake. Activation of the PNS slows heart rate, decreases blood pressure, increases digestive activity, and promotes relaxation. The PNS is a crucial component of the autonomic nervous system (ANS) that promotes relaxation and conserves energy. However, when this freeze response has become overactive or is not working collaboratively with the other parts of the brain, these recurring imbalances in PNS activity can contribute to a variety of health concerns. When the brake is on for too long, it's the opposite of being alert and engaged – the overloaded PNS can feel paralyzing.

Again, people stuck in this state, with the parking brake locked on, will also seek relief at almost any cost.

Symmetry versus Asymmetry

Your brain wants to operate in symmetry or with balance. Like the gas and brake of your car, it wants to work in harmony.

Asymmetry, however, means the brain is physically out of balance, and one part of the CNS is dominant and in charge. This imbalance can present as unintended or undesirable behavior.

If the brain is stuck in a sympathetic state, like the gas pedal has a brick stuck on it, this person is in a constant fight or flight state. Behaviorally, this may show up as yelling, arguing, slamming doors, punching walls, aggression, or even fleeing out of the house (fight OR flight). It can feel like the person's state of mind and reasoning have been hijacked and they are no longer feeling in control.

Alternatively, if the brain is stuck in an overwhelmed parasympathetic state—the parking brake is fully engaged—this person is in a freeze response. Behaviorally this may show up by wanting to isolate, procrastination, being unable to engage socially, refusing to leave the comfort and safety of home, having difficulty managing hygiene, feeling numb, an inability to make eye contact, wearing clothing that helps the person to hide, like a hoodie or hat, to disappear emotionally. They are essentially curling up in a ball to make themselves *small* in an attempt to disappear or become invisible. At the very least, this sends a message to people in the room not to bother or engage with them.

Either of these patterns or behaviors occur because the brain perceives it is under attack, being threatened, or it has experienced chronic stress or trauma. Remember that the brain only focuses on its primary job—keeping you alive. Despite negative consequences, the brain takes over the response and will not relinquish control regardless of logic, desire to change, or having remorse for actions. Your safety and survival are hard-wired in the brain.

Your nervous system is phenomenal when operating correctly. If a burglar breaks into your home, you want to quickly react and act in a fight or flight response. If you discover the loud noise was just a neighbor, or maybe a pesky raccoon, you want your brain to realize that there is no danger so it can return to a relaxed, harmonious, and balanced state.

When the brain is faced with a life-threatening situation, the CNS will kick in or react. If the event is perceived to be extreme, the CNS will react in an extreme way in an attempt to keep you safe and alive. The nervous system can be overwhelmed by stress (trauma), which results in the CNS staying stuck even ***after*** the traumatic event has subsided long ago. The event does not have to be life-threatening to create this imbalance in the CNS. It can also be caused by chronic stress, grief, emotional pain, physical pain, hardship, or even a perceived attack, and more.

Give Me Relief!

Now, let's introduce a substance or behavior to the brain and nervous system conversation.

If a brain is stuck and the gas pedal or the brake is fully engaged, you will very likely be struggling. Sleep may be impaired with the adrenaline surging throughout your body. Maybe as soon as your head hits the pillow and it's quiet with no distractions, your mind and thoughts take off. You may feel annoyed, fearful, panicked, constantly vigilant, confrontational, convinced that something catastrophic is going to happen, restless, agitated, anxious, overwhelmed, buzzing, shaky, helpless and hopeless, have a queasy stomach, and more.

You are emotionally dysregulated and physically exhausted.

Consuming a substance (like alcohol or marijuana) or engaging in a behavior (like shopping, gaming, binge-watching, or emotional eating) gives you a reprieve from these overwhelming and unbearable physical or emotional states for a brief period. You have temporarily changed how your brain is functioning, and you may feel better, maybe even happy. Your brain quickly learns that you need more of that substance or behavior to get relief. What it can't predict is that this solution will only bring about temporary solace and will create many more problems.

It doesn't take a neuroscientist to figure out what will most likely happen — you're going to seek relief again and again and again, despite negative consequences. Your brain doesn't care about long-term consequences. It only wants relief from the current pain and dysfunction.

Dr. Gabor Maté is a Canadian physician, author, and public speaker known for his work on the impact of trauma and stress on physical and mental health. Dr. Maté argues that addictions, such as drug abuse, alcoholism, and gambling, are rooted in childhood trauma and emotional pain.

> The question is not why the addiction, but why the pain?
> - Dr. Gabor Maté

Dr. Maté believes that the root cause of addiction lies in the brain's reward system.

Dr. Maté also stresses that addiction is often a way for individuals to cope with unresolved emotional pain. Many people who struggle with addiction have experienced trauma, abuse, lack of safety, stability, or neglect in their childhood. They may use substances or behaviors as a way to numb their emotional pain or to escape from unregulated emotions or crushing reality.

Dr. Daniel Amen and Amen Clinics

Dr. Daniel Amen is a renowned psychiatrist and brain-imaging specialist, pioneering the use of functional brain imaging in efforts to more accurately diagnose and treat mental health disorders, behavioral disorders, and addictions.

Dr. Amen is the founder of Amen Clinics, which utilizes SPECT (single-photon emission computerized tomography) scans to enhance understanding and treatment of addictions. SPECT measures blood flow and activity in the brain and shows areas of the brain with healthy activity, too much activity, and too little activity. These scans reveal crucial abnormalities in key behavior-related brain areas, such as the frontal lobes, in substance abusers. This brain imaging is invaluable as it visually demonstrates that underlying brain dysfunction is the primary reason why individuals experience addiction. Unhealthy brain activity is also associated with an increased risk of relapse. In addition, SPECT scans reveal the physical impact of drugs and alcohol on the brain, emphasizing that addiction detrimentally affects crucial brain functions necessary for recovery and a fulfilling life.

He has shown that addiction is a brain-related issue that requires a personalized approach to treatment. Individuals can achieve lasting recovery and improved overall health and wellbeing through specific tailored recommendations and lifestyle interventions by identifying and addressing underlying brain imbalances and emotional issues.

Dr. Amen's approach to addiction treatment emphasizes individualized care based on a comprehensive evaluation that includes brain imaging. His holistic strategy also integrates biological, psychological, social, and spiritual elements, focusing on healing the entire person rather than just addressing the addiction (think of the Iceberg model we presented in Chapter 1 going to a deeper layer beyond just the addiction is critical to creating lasting recovery).

A Balanced Brain—Using Technology to Speed Up Recovery

Cereset is a private neurotechnology company headquartered in Scottsdale, Arizona. Lee Gerdes, CEO, developed a noninvasive neurotechnology that is available throughout the US and globally.

As discussed earlier in this chapter, when a brain is imbalanced (asymmetric), a person's behavior can be negatively impacted. It has nothing to do with a character defect, lack of willpower, or even forgiveness. It is all about an imbalanced nervous system that can drive certain negative behaviors.

Cereset's noninvasive technology supports the brain in relaxing and rebalancing or resetting itself for optimal regulation. This is an *inside-out* approach, which we will explore later in this book.

In turn, this is helpful for reducing cravings and triggers that are associated with addiction. Research suggests that addiction can cause changes in brain function and connectivity. Rebalancing brain function can then help to restore balance and improve quality of life. With Cereset, the results happen within days. The efficacy is a result of supporting the brain to relax itself so the brain can self-regulate and rebalance on its own terms.

> Some people may continue to see themselves as inferior to the guy who bullied them in school, while their brains adapt to this "reality". If we instead chose to believe that all humans are unique and equal – and we have the power to make society fairer – this will change our brains too. It is a clear example of how attitudes can alter both brains and behaviour.
>
> - Jordan Peterson, PhD

The Brain-First Approach

It is critical to understand that the brain drives behavior. The brain is your master hard drive that controls how you think, feel, and what you do.

The point of this chapter is to highlight the importance of acceptance to adapt and implement new ideas for overcoming addictions and realizing sustainable recovery. Because of this, Actualized Recovery encourages a fully integrative approach to long-term recovery that embraces the most recent and progressive scientific research.

In all other sciences and medical practices, focus is placed on the sick organ that is driving the illness, preferably with an integrative approach. The title is Brain-FIRST, not Brain-ONLY. Actualized Recovery recognizes that life is complex and integrated. However, it is about viewing all integrated solutions through the lens of what optimizes brain function.

Your brain is an organ that holds within it the power for your life to flourish. Most legitimate professional, scientific, and academic groups in modern times—who have studied addictions and recovery—all agree and connect addictive patterns with the brain. Without acknowledging this widely accepted fact, any path to recovery you embark on that does not accept this will likely have short-lived results.

It is time to look at all forms of recovery from a brain-first paradigm.

It's not about willpower. It's not about a higher power. ***It's all about brain power.***

Chapter 3

It's Not a Lack of Willpower

Like it or not, your brain drives your behavior.

- Lee Gerdes

Correlation Between the Brain and Behavior

Families with a loved one who has been affected by Alzheimer's or other dementia will tell you it's a sickening and dreadful decline of the person's mental and physical capacities. It is a heart-wrenching process to witness and for the person to live through. These neurodegenerative diseases slowly ravage the memory of everything that truly matters and create catastrophic cognitive decline, stealing dignity as it eventually robs the person of every independence of life, including the ability to recognize those they love, to speak, to independently eat, bathe, dress, or use a toilet. They lose the ability to have freedom and sovereignty over their own life, slowly fading into an isolated world that has no resemblance to the vibrant soul who accomplished so much.

We know this only too well, as both of us (Susan and Dave) witnessed our beloved mothers disappear into the silent confusion of their brain's inability to remember or communicate.

The point we wish to highlight is that Alzheimer's or other dementias negatively impact brain function. They ravage the actual organ itself. As the brain becomes impaired, so does the person and their ability to live an autonomous and full life.

Today's incredible neurotechnologies allow us to see how the brain—the hard drive—is negatively impacted and changed by trauma. Magnetic Resonance Imaging (MRI) and SPECT imaging reveal the deterioration of brain function.

There are two key takeaways from modern understanding of these neurological conditions. First, this loss of a *person* is not a result of the mind. Second, this loss of a *person* is certainly not a lack of willpower. In the case of Alzheimer's or other dementias, the deterioration is caused by a poorly functioning and degenerating brain.

> You don't have to look any deeper than Alzheimer's and other dementias to understand there is a direct correlation between the brain and behavior.

This is a book about recovery, and the same principles and recommendations apply to keep your brain functioning optimally and to avoid cognitive impairment as you age. We wish that we had known decades ago what we know now to have been able to keep our moms with us in mind, body, and spirit.

The Brain-Behavior Connection

The brain-behavior connection is like the relationship between a sophisticated software program and the computer processor it runs on. Think of your brain as a highly advanced processor, constantly receiving and interpreting data from sensory inputs like touch, taste, sight, smell, and sound. This data is then analyzed, leading to responses and actions. For instance, if your hand encounters a hot surface, the brain instantly processes this sensation and triggers a reflex to pull away, prioritizing safety.

This complex interaction governs every aspect of human behavior, from spontaneous reactions to deliberate choices like opting for a healthy snack over junk food. It's like a complex algorithm making real-time decisions based on incoming data. This connection is crucial in shaping not only your physical responses, but also your emotions, thoughts, and dreams. It's the foundation of your interactions with the world, enabling you to engage in activities ranging from athletic endeavors to your relationships and wealth (or debt).

This also includes your choices. Where you go, what you do, and who you choose to hang out with are all brain-driven. Where do you go after work—the bar or the gym? Who do you hang out with—smokers or yogis? Your brain drives all choices. Neuroscience and psychology professionals agree that if you want a different outcome, then you need to consider how to reprogram your brain. And you can!

Behavior, by definition, is an action, activity, or process that can be observed and measured. Behavior is how people or animals act or react, often in response to what's happening around them or their feelings. It's not just about what someone does, but also what they choose not to do. Whether it's talking, playing, or even just sitting still, all these actions are examples of behavior. Simply stated, a behavior is defined by a person's actions or inactions.

> Your brain is your own personal hard drive, or master control center. It is your brain that drives everything you do, and don't do.

Intentions do not correlate with behavior. A person's intentions are difficult to observe or measure because they are subjective. Here's an example: when driving a car, your intention might be to stay within the speed limit. It comes down to a simple question of whether you do or do not stay within the speed limit. What you do is quantifiable, but your intention is not. You choose the action.

Inaction is also a choice and can be an equally powerful behavioral pattern. Not showing up to work or school or staying in bed all day is a behavioral choice. The choice of *not to act* can be observed and measured and does have a consequence or a result.

Viktor Frankl was a famous Jewish Austrian psychiatrist, neurologist, author, and World War II Holocaust survivor. He authored *Man's Search for Meaning*, one of the most influential books of the 20th century. This is a profound exploration of the impact of helplessness, and the human spirit's resilience and quest for purpose or meaning.

Frankl developed many concepts in the field of psychology that are widely practiced today. He referred to one of his core concepts as *logotherapy*. It emphasizes finding meaning in life as the primary motivational force for individuals. It focuses on the future and on our ability to endure hardship and suffering through a sense of purpose and by finding meaning in life events, especially in challenging circumstances.

Frankl also observed that when fellow Holocaust prisoners lost hope of ever being rescued, deep-seated helplessness would set in, and their spirit to endure would evaporate. The result was their candle would go out, typically within a few hours.

Frankl greatly influenced the understanding of choice and behavior. He is credited with developing Logotherapy, which teaches us that "Between stimulus and response lies a space. In that space lie our power and freedom to choose a response. In our response lies our growth and our happiness." This space (or gap) is the ability to choose our reaction (note: there is a debate as to who wrote this. Some people have credited Stephen Covey, but he has denied being the author. The most recent and accurate research attributes this quote to Frankl).

This concept has long been accepted in psychology and human performance. We all have the power of choice.

We are not powerless over any external or internal stimuli. Regardless of the circumstance we may find ourselves in, we have the power to choose our responses and actions.

This can be both freeing and scary. Frankl's teachings mean we are fully and completely accountable and responsible for our choices and actions. Regardless of how we perceive an event, there is a gap—a moment in time where we are able to choose our response. We can choose to be a victim of life and continue to drift or embrace having extreme ownership of our lives.

> Between stimulus and response lies a space. In that space lies our growth and our happiness.
>
> - Viktor Frankl

When looking at self-destructive choices (behaviors), there is more choice than one may think. Once someone initiates or consumes an addictive behavior like gambling, shopping, or using a substance, it can be reasonably argued that they may now be in a powerless state because the horses are out of the barn, so to speak. In other words, once the behavior starts, it may be too late to implement choice as the brain has now been hijacked. This person is in a reactive state.

But what if the gap or space is not after they start drinking (gambling, eating, etc.) ***but before***? For example, what if that gap is ***before*** the person enters the bar? What if multiple gaps represent a series of choices that lead them to walk into the bar in the first place? What if that gap happens hours before when *drinking friends* invite someone out to the bar? What if, in that split-second gap, the person chooses to meet friends at the gym instead? It seems logical that making a different choice (not going to the bar) will have a very different outcome or behavior. What if that person created new friendships that didn't even involve drinking?

We all have this power. It is the power to make a choice in the gap between an internal or external stimulus and our response.

Despite living through the hell of the Holocaust and its evil brutality, Frankl's theory was tested again and again in the war camps. The pain and suffering he and so many others endured is inconceivable. Yet he maintained that he, and only he, got to choose his response to starvation, to torture and torment, to psychological and spiritual abuse. In his words, "in that space lie our power and freedom."

Coaching Tip:

We encourage you to pause for a moment. Yes, stop reading. Reflect on Frankl's teachings (read the above paragraph a second time). Let it set in with you. Consider and apply this knowledge to any challenge (or addiction) you are struggling with. Frankl's teachings show us that none of us are powerless. You are not powerless. You do have the power to choose your response to anything. With that, you become empowered with greater resilience, strength, and hope.

Woundology or Trauma Attraction

Caroline Myss, a 5-time New York Times best selling author, insightfully wrote the book *Why People Don't Heal and How They Can*. In her book, she introduces the concept of "woundology" to help understand how individuals often relate to their past traumas and hardships. According to Myss, it's common for people to identify themselves primarily through the lens of their past wounds and sufferings. This can be seen when individuals consistently bring up their past traumas in conversations, using them to gain sympathy or explain their current life situation. This also gives them access to a group of people or a culture who have experienced similar trauma and who also identify themselves by their past traumatic experiences.

Woundology is like carrying a backpack filled with old, heavy rocks representing our past hurts and traumas. Some people get so used to the weight of this backpack that they feel it's a part of who they are. They always talk about these rocks and use them to explain why they act a certain way or why things don't go well for them.

In essence, people can become so tied to their identity as a *victim* of their circumstances that it hinders their ability to grow and move beyond their past. This perpetual state of identifying with one's wounds can create a sense of powerlessness, making individuals feel that they are constantly at the mercy of their past experiences.

Myss advocates for a more empowering approach. She suggests that acknowledging our past traumas is just the first step. The real work lies in moving beyond them, which involves shifting our focus from what happened to us, to how we can grow from those experiences. This doesn't mean ignoring the pain or the impact of past events, but rather learning to see them as part of a larger journey toward personal growth and self-understanding. By doing so, individuals can embrace their potential and strength rather than being defined solely by their past wounds.

This encourages a shift from a mindset of victimhood to one of acceptance and growth, promoting resilience and the ability to face life's challenges with a more constructive and hopeful perspective. You can acknowledge your tough times without letting them hold you back. This paradigm shift is about seeing your struggles as opportunities with rich lessons by which to grow, not as anchors.

Habits, Choices, and Behaviors

There is a naturally strong desire to learn more about developing habits for two reasons. First is the effort to help people make the choices they desire. The second is to help people live a life of abundance and thrive.

Understanding how habits are formed provides the key to helping change those patterns, choices, and behaviors for the desired outcome.

Let's Geek Out

Neurons – You have approximately 100 billion neurons in your brain. That's more neurons in your brain than stars in our galaxy. A neuron is a cell in the brain that's like a tiny messenger that works at incredible speed. It sends and receives messages. This intricate network of neurons and their connections is the foundation of all brain activities, including thought, emotion, sensation, and motor control. The incredible complexity and adaptability of these neural networks enable the brain to learn, remember, and adapt to new experiences.

Synapse – A synaptic connection is like a tiny, specialized meeting point between two neurons in the brain. Imagine two people passing a note across a small gap – that's what happens at a synapse. This connection allows the neurons to communicate, passing messages that control everything from our thoughts and feelings to our movements. Each synaptic connection is part of a vast network in our brain, making it possible for us to learn, remember, and interact with the world.

Neural pathway – A neural pathway, or neural circuit, is like a well-trodden hiking trail through a forest, but in your brain. It's a series of connected neurons that communicate with each other to send specific messages. Each time you think, feel, or do something, you're activating a particular pathway. Just like walking the same trail repeatedly makes it more defined, the more you use a neural pathway, the stronger and more efficient it becomes. This is why habits and skills become easier over time – your brain is getting better at sending signals along these familiar 'trails'. These pathways are crucial for learning, memory, and forming habits.

Hebb's Law or Hebbian Theory

Donald O. Hebb (1904-1985) has been referred to as the "father of neuropsychology." Hebb was a Canadian psychologist whose contribution to both the field of psychology and neuroscience has become a cornerstone in human behavior and learning.

> The more a neuron fires,
> the stronger it wires.
> - Hebb's Law

Hebbian Theory, commonly known as Hebb's Law, explains how learning and habit-forming occur within the human brain. His theory was based on neurological cell assembly or synaptic connections.

A synapse is a link between nerve cells; these connections help us learn and adapt to the world around us. When a neuron fires (activates), it creates a synaptic connection with another neuron. Here is an example: when we repeat an action, like throwing a ball, the more we toss the ball, the easier it becomes and the more proficient we are at this function. The main reason for this increase in proficiency is what we call Hebb's Law: "the more a neuron fires the stronger it wires." This repeated action creates a neural pathway that makes it easier over time to replicate this behavior.

In short, if neuron 'A' repeatedly fires with neuron 'B', a change occurs, improving and strengthening how the two cells communicate or 'fire.' If repeated over and over, this connection will become more efficient, faster, and more predominant. The phrase "neurons (cells) that fire together, wire together" has been commonly used to describe this synaptic connection theory presented by Hebb.

Learning to ride a bicycle is a very complex task. Your brain must coordinate balance, pedaling, steering, and awareness simultaneously, which involves many different neurons firing simultaneously.

This is why its good to start with a tricycle. Then graduate to a two-wheeler with training wheels. Eventually, a child is ready to take the training wheels off, but for safety, a parent typically grabs the seat and charges along with the child to avoid a significant crash. And then in one instant...you can see it, you can feel it....YES....off they go. Wobbly at first. Maybe ten feet. Then twenty-five feet. Within days, they are cruising the entire neighborhood.

So what exactly just happened?

Each time you practice, the neural pathways involved in biking are activated. According to Hebb's Law, because these neurons are firing at the same time, the connections between them strengthen. The more you do it, the easier it becomes. This is like carving a smoother, more direct path through a dense forest. The more you practice, the stronger and more efficient these pathways become, making riding the bike feel more natural and automatic. Eventually, you can ride without consciously thinking about each action, thanks to the reinforced neural pathways created by repeated practice.

Hebb's Law—A Double-Edged Sword

Hebb has given the world a model to view and understand synaptic connections, which essentially is how our brain 'learns.' The result is that there is a multitude of practical implications for people. In short, the synaptic connection hypothesis Hebb has presented can be a double-edged sword when it comes to human behavior.

Hebb's Law, often summarized as "neurons that fire together, wire together," is akin to brushing your teeth with your dominant hand. Just as using your dominant hand to brush your teeth feels natural and effortless due to years of repeated practice, Hebb's Law explains how frequently used neural pathways in the brain become stronger and more efficient. Each time you brush with your dominant hand, you reinforce the neural connections that make this task feel automatic.

However, attempting to brush your teeth with your non-dominant hand is like forging a new path through a dense, uncharted forest. It takes more time, energy, and focus to complete the same task and is a lot messier. Initially, it feels awkward and clumsy because the neural pathways for this activity are underdeveloped. But, just as a path in a forest becomes clearer and easier to traverse with repeated use, so too do the neural connections in your brain strengthen with practice. Over time, what once felt awkward can become more natural and skilled, demonstrating the incredible adaptability of the brain according to Hebbian theory. This metaphor illustrates the essence of Hebb's Law and emphasizes the power of neuroplasticity and our brain's capacity to learn and adapt through repetition and practice.

The big take-away is that neurons fire and rewire by 'action'. Doing (an action) causes your neurons to fire and the more you repeat this action the stronger or more dominant they become. You can not accomplish this by knowledge alone. Watching a video tutorial, or having a dentist explain how to brush your teeth, or reading a book will not create new neural pathways.

Conversely, when a person repeats a negative pattern or behavior, they will also be creating stronger synaptic connections in the same manner. Repetition will again make the synaptic firing more wired, or more dominant, making a negative behavior a more likely pattern.

We will say it again – the phrase "neurons that fire together wire together" aptly describes this learning process. This has a direct impact on human behavior, whether it be positive or negative.

The more times you grab a morning coffee, go outside, and light a cigarette, the stronger you are hard-wiring this into your brain. The more times you repeat this behavior, the more dominant it becomes. So, if your goal is to stop smoking, it is wise then to change the entire pattern and repeat a new, different action. Because if you pour your coffee and go outside to your favorite perch, your brain will be more likely to crave that cigarette as part of the pattern. It's less about the cigarette and more about rewiring your brain and creating a new neural pathway for a brighter future.

Hebbian theory has lasting and profound implications regarding neuroplasticity, learning, forging habits, and human behavior. Change takes time. And it takes effort. You may, no, you will, feel awkward at first, like brushing your teeth with your non-dominant hand. The key to creating different outcomes is to 'do' something and repeat this action consistently over time.

Habituation

Habits are formed in the brain through a process called "habituation." Habituation involves gradually strengthening neural connections (Hebb's Law) between specific stimuli, actions, and rewards.

When a behavior is continually repeated, the brain gradually forms a 'habit loop' that consists of three components:

1. Cue: A specific stimulus, situation, or context that triggers the behavior.
2. Routine: The actual behavior or action performed in response to the cue.
3. Reward: The positive outcome or consequence that reinforces the behavior and makes it more likely to be repeated in the future.

The formation of a habit occurs when the brain gradually learns to associate the cue, routine, and reward together. Each time the habit loop is activated within the brain, the neural connections between the cue, routine, and reward are strengthened, making the behavior more automatic and less conscious.

Neurotransmitters, such as dopamine, also play a role in habit formation. Dopamine is released in response to rewarding experiences and reinforces the neural connections involved in the habit loop, making the behavior involuntary or automatic.

Over time, habits become deeply ingrained in the brain and can be difficult (but possible) to break. This is because the neural connections involved in the habit loop become so strong that they can override conscious decision-making (willpower) processes. However, habits can be changed through intentional effort and repetition of new behaviors, which gradually weaken the old neural connections and forge new ones, which, over time, become stronger.

Neural Pruning

The simple phrase "use it or lose it" accurately describes the brain's process of eliminating unnecessary connections.

Neural pruning is the brain's process of eliminating weak or unnecessary connections between neurons. This helps to streamline the brain's neural network and make it more efficient. It happens most prolifically during childhood and adolescence, as the brain is still developing.

Neural pruning is like cleaning your closet and getting rid of old clothes you no longer need. By eliminating weak or unnecessary connections, the brain can optimize its neural network and improve communication between neurons.

We've all experienced neural pruning. If you stop doing an activity or a habit for an extended period of time, that behavior becomes less dominant, and the new pattern becomes the dominant behavior. It feels difficult and uncomfortable initially because the brain has been hardwired. It takes conscious effort over time to undo a habit. Think of writing with your non-dominant hand – it can be messy.

If you want to change a habit or pattern, it demands consistent action. Over time, the effort required diminishes as the new pattern becomes more dominant. Consistent action over time creates success by leveraging the power of Hebb's Law.

In conclusion, the more a behavior is repeated, the stronger the firing neurons develop and the more dominant the habit becomes. In essence, every person is, knowingly or unknowingly, training their brain with their actions.

> What syncs in the brain,
> links in the brain.
> - Dr. Joe Dispenza

Since our goal is to profoundly impact people, helping them realize positive change and lasting recovery, it is imperative to grasp Hebb's Law and leverage it in any modality designed to create change or enhance human performance.

An Impaired Brain Loses the Ability to Reason

AA and 12-step programs first have you admit that you are powerless over alcohol, gambling, gaming, shopping, etc. If you accept that as truth, meaning that you are 'powerless,' then a logical question is, ***how*** did you become powerless? What exactly has caused you to lose your ability to choose?

What happens to have you surrender all sense of reason, do things that may hurt people that you love, put your life and others at risk, squander resources, break promises, perhaps even break the law, and have dire, irreversible consequences?

Is this a moral failing? Is it a biological failing? Is it a psychological disruption? Is it caused by genetics? Is it a spiritual defect?

Your sense of reasoning resides mainly in the frontal lobe of your brain, and if that area has become unable to reason, meaning to analyze information to predict a possible negative outcome, you'll make many bad decisions. The frontal lobe has been nicknamed the 'executive manager' because this is where you make decisions. Anything a person does that involves thinking, choosing, acting, reasoning, judgment, decision-making, and more is processed in the frontal lobe. When brain function is imbalanced or asymmetric, processing and decision-making are typically flawed or impaired.

The human brain does not mature until approximately 25 years of age. This is when a person has greater cognitive capacity to understand the correlation between actions and consequences. Ever wonder why car rental companies refuse to rent to anyone under the age of 25? It's because the insurance underwriters grasp the importance of a fully developed brain, specifically the frontal lobe. Accident rates drop off sharply at this age, making them more responsible drivers.

What if the toxicity of the substances is one of the contributors that can cause your brain not to be able to be reasonable or reasoned with? What if many things impede your sense of logic or reality?

The next question is, what can be done to restore autonomy and a sense of reason? Well, how about we ask the rats.

Rat Park – It's Where All the Happy Rats Live

The Rat Park experiment was a study conducted by psychologist Bruce Alexander and his colleagues in the late 1970s and early 1980s. The experiment was designed to explore the role of the environment in addiction and substance abuse.

Alexander and his colleagues housed rats in two different environments in the experiment. One group of rats was housed in standard laboratory cages, while the other group was housed in a larger, more upgraded environment called "Rat Park." Rat Park was a spacious enclosure that included toys, tunnels, and other rats for social interaction.

Both groups of rats were given access to two water bottles - one containing plain water and the other containing a solution of morphine or heroin. The researchers found that the rats housed in standard laboratory cages strongly preferred the drug-laced water, consumed it at a much higher rate than the plain water, and had a much higher mortality rate. In contrast, the rats housed in Rat Park consumed much less of the drug-laced water and showed a weaker preference for it.

The researchers concluded that the rats in standard laboratory cages were more likely to become addicted to the drug because they were living in a lonely and distressing environment. We can also point out that these rats have lost their sense of reasoning or sound decision-making ability. In contrast, the rats in Rat Park had access to a more fulfilling environment with opportunities for social interaction, exercise, and play. This environment provided the rats with more positive sources of pleasure, reducing their interest and dependence on the drug-laced water.

The Rat Park experiment challenged the prevailing view at the time that the chemical properties of drugs primarily caused addiction. Instead, the study suggested that environmental factors, such as social interaction and environmental enhancement, play a critical role in addiction and substance abuse.

The findings of the Rat Park experiment have since been supported by additional studies, suggesting that how we live can have a significant impact on addiction and substance abuse in humans as well as animals. These findings have important implications for addiction treatment and prevention, emphasizing the importance of creating positive social and environmental conditions for individuals struggling with addiction.

These findings were revolutionary in the field of addiction. The Rat Park study changed everything we once believed about addiction or SUD.

Here is one of the most powerful questions not being asked in today's addiction recovery field: Even with all of this research evidence, what do we do as a society? It's still common and accepted to shame, blame, and then isolate people with addiction problems. In essence, we create a punitive environment, either imposed by society or family or often self-imposed and then wonder why people don't get better.

Neuroscience and behavioral sciences teach us that isolation and a desolate environment negatively impact the brain in both size and function. This darkens the spirit, bringing on a more profound sense of hopelessness.

When the world can approach an addiction or limiting behavior from a *brain-first* perspective, it alleviates all shame, blame, and social shunning. We must begin by restoring the person's ability to reason by rebooting or resetting the frontal lobe of the brain, enhancing the ability to make better decisions.

To attain this goal requires leveraging and integrating the newest findings in applied neuroscience. This direction is vital to release any outdated stigma. Accepting and understanding that the brain itself is the master of behavior creates the opportunity to regain power and reclaim control of our own life.

When a person has a heart or liver that is not functioning properly, the person's health and wellbeing suffer, and their

> Consider the compelling hope and opportunity for lasting full recovery and wellbeing when treatment and therapy embrace a brain-first approach to thriving.

life may be in peril. Once diagnosed, the doctors and medical specialists immediately look at the impaired organ to create a treatment plan for the dysfunctional or ill organ. There is no shame involved. It is viewed and accepted as a sick organ requiring effective and targeted treatment.

We contend that an addiction or behavioral weakness is merely a symptom of a person seeking relief from pain and/or trauma, which has resulted in neuro-asymmetry. In an effort of desperation, people seek and consume all sorts of substances or engage in negative self-destructive behaviors simply to get relief from their pain, regardless of the long-term costs to their life, relationships, careers, family, finances, and more.

Let's end the shame and social stigma of addictions or SUD, and self-sabotaging habits. It's time to embrace science and the power of your brain to change.

Chapter 4

Brain-First

Your brain is responsible for everything you think, feel, and do.

Your Actual Brain—Human IT Hardware

Your brain is at the center of your being. Your identity is formed and upheld in your brain. It is your personal bio-computer controlling who you are and how you navigate this world.

It weighs approximately three pounds, has the consistency of soft tofu, and is comprised of over 100 billion neurons. Neurons are brain cells that transmit and receive nerve impulses and form all communication between the brain and body. You have more neurons in your brain than there are stars in the universe. These 100 billion neurons have trillions of neural connections, all working in a magically choreographed sequence, keeping you alive and, if it has leftover energy, living the life that matters most to you.

Your brain has many critical and intricate functions, and its primary role is keeping everything in your body working well for your survival. It is a highly complex organ that controls your breathing, hydration, organ function, body temperature, immune response, touch, motor skills, vision, sleep, comprehension, memory, speech, language, digestion, excretion, and every other process and nuance that regulates your body. This balance of life-sustaining efforts is called homeostasis. The brain also influences your thoughts, your emotional response, what and who you're attracted to, and your capacity for intelligence.

Now that you have some knowledge of the physical brain, let's explore the difference between the brain and the mind. Science and psychology have wrestled with this distinction since the time of Aristotle. Recent advancements in neurotechnology (technology used to measure and map how your brain is functioning in real time) is showing us that there is a significant difference between the mind and the brain.

The Mind—Human IT Software

Your mind is not your physical brain. Your mind is independent yet connected with your brain.

Dr. Carolyn Leaf is a neuroscientist whose passion is to help people see the power of the mind to change the function of the brain, control chaotic thinking, and find mental peace. Backed by clinical research and various case studies, Dr. Leaf's research tells us that the mind is an energy flow, comprising a stream of nonconscious activity as we sleep and streams of conscious and unconscious activity when we are awake. Her clinical findings define the mind as being characterized by energetic actions, including feeling (emotions), thinking, and the ability to choose.

> The brain is the physiology (function). The mind is the psychology (mental characteristics).

Mindfulness Practice, Cognitive Behavior Therapy (CBT) Neuro-Linguistic Programming (NLP), Eye Movement Desensitization and Reprocessing (EMDR) Therapy, and so many more therapeutic modalities are designed to change how the mind processes.

When defining the brain versus the mind, we often use an IT metaphor: your brain is your hard drive (as introduced earlier) while your mind is the software. However, we'd like to share another metaphor that depicts this complex relationship with ease.

Imagine the brain as a grand, intricate orchestra, composed of various sections like strings, brass, woodwinds, and percussion. Each section represents different parts of the brain, responsible for various functions like memory, emotion, reasoning, and movement. The musicians in the orchestra are like the neurons in the brain, each playing their part, communicating and coordinating to create a harmonious symphony.

Now, picture the mind as the music that this orchestra produces. It's not something you can touch or see, but it's a beautiful, complex result of all the instruments (or brain parts) working together. The mind encompasses our thoughts, feelings, memories, and consciousness – the melody, harmony, and rhythm arising from the brain's physical structure and activity.

In this story, the conductor of the orchestra symbolizes the intricate interplay between different brain regions. The conductor ensures that all sections come together in synchrony, creating a cohesive piece of music just as the brain integrates various inputs and processes to produce the harmony of the mind.

So, the relationship between the brain and the mind is like that of an orchestra and its music. The brain is the physical entity (the orchestra with its musicians and instruments), and the mind is the resulting, intangible experience (the music that fills the concert hall), felt and experienced in a way that transcends the mere physical presence of the instruments.

Your Central Nervous System

As we talked about in Chapter 2, there are two significant parts of our Central Nervous System (CNS); the Sympathetic Nervous System (SNS), and the Parasympathetic Nervous System (PNS).

The sympathetic nervous system is the fight or flight response to distress (whether the danger is real or perceived). It's like a fire alarm in a building. When a potential threat or stressful situation arises, it acts like the alarm going off, quickly alerting and mobilizing the entire 'building'—your body. It sends signals to increase heart rate, expand airways, and release stored energy, preparing the body to either face the challenge or escape it. This response is like the alarm preparing its occupants for urgent action, whether it's an evacuation or immediate response to danger, ensuring readiness and rapid reaction in high-stress situations. This is a wonderful system to ensure our safety and survival.

However, a serious problem can arise when the sympathetic nervous system (SNS) becomes overly active and stays on 'all the time'. It's like an alarm system that keeps going off unnecessarily, putting the body in a constant state of high alert. This can be compared to living in a house where the alarm is always sounding, creating a continuous sense of urgency and stress. In such a situation, the body remains in its "fight or flight" mode for too long. This constant state of arousal can lead to a variety of issues like increased blood pressure, stress, anxiety, anger or rage, disappearing, running away, and difficulty sleeping. And if a persons SNS remains in a state of high alert take a wild guess what they are going to look for? Relief!

We often call it self-medication, whether that's in the form of alcohol or other substances or behaviors. They seek relief to give the brain and nervous system a sense of temporary calm. So, you better believe this person is going to seek a substance or behavior for internal relief.

The parasympathetic nervous system (PNS) can be described as the caretaker of a restful garden retreat. Just as a caretaker maintains a garden that promotes growth and restoration, the PNS helps the body relax, recover, and rejuvenate after periods of stress or activity. It's like gently watering the plants, ensuring they're nourished and the environment is calm and peaceful, encouraging a state of tranquility. This system lowers the heart rate, eases breathing, and stimulates digestion, much like a caretaker ensures that every part of the garden is tended to, promoting a serene and healthful atmosphere. It's the force that says, "Slow down, rest, and rebuild," after the excitement and rush, ensuring balance and wellbeing.

Yet another challenge arises if the PNS takes charge full-time or becomes locked-on. When the parasympathetic nervous system becomes overly dominant, it's like a garden caretaker who overwaters the plants and keeps them in constant shade. While some rest and nourishment are good, too much can hinder the garden's vitality. Instead of thriving, the plants become weak and unable to withstand external conditions. Similarly, if the parasympathetic system is dominant and in-charge, the body may become too relaxed, leading to lethargy, low energy levels, and a decreased ability to respond to necessary stimuli, even complete isolation. When the PNS is always engaged this drives people also to seek relief which is oftentimes found through a substance or behavior. But any relief is short-term, leaving the brain wanting more. Just like a garden needs a balance of sun and shade, water and space to grow, our bodies need a balance between rest (parasympathetic) and activity (sympathetic) to function optimally.

Physiology Drives Psychology

The statement "physiology drives psychology" underlines that our physical state and biological processes significantly influence our mental state and psychological experiences. Essentially, it means that the condition and functioning of our body can shape our thoughts, emotions, and behaviors.

This concept underscores the deep interconnection between our physical bodies and our mental states. It connects that our thoughts and experiences do not just influence our mental health and psychological processes but are also deeply rooted in our biological functioning.

For instance, hormonal imbalances can affect mood, a lack of sleep can impact cognitive abilities, and stress can trigger psychological disturbances. This concept supports the notion that to understand and treat psychological issues, one should also consider the underlying physiological factors. It's like saying that the foundation of a house (physiology) affects the shape and stability of the structure built on top of it (psychology). If the foundation is not stable or is in a state of dis-ease, it will inevitably impact the entire structure. When you're exhausted or hungry your concentration, focus, memory and your emotional regulation will suffer. Your family may notice you're grumpy or angry (known as being hangry). This shows how your physical state can change your mood, your thinking, and your overall performance.

The same goes for exercise - when you're physically active, you feel better mentally. When you exercise, your brain releases several types of endorphins, which are chemicals produced by the body to relieve stress and pain. They are often referred to as "feel-good" hormones because of their ability to produce a sense of wellbeing or even euphoria, sometimes known as the "runner's high."

These endorphins act as natural painkillers and mood elevators, reducing the perception of pain and triggering positive feelings in the body. Regular exercise has also been shown to enhance brain function and stimulate brain growth. This is why regular physical activity is often recommended for managing stress, anxiety, and depression.

In treatments and therapy, this connection means that taking care of your physical health is also important for your mental health. Practices like yoga and breathwork are good for your body and your mind. They help you feel better overall by ensuring your physical and mental health are in harmony.

So, "physiology drives psychology" is a way of saying that to be mentally healthy, it's important to take care of your physical health. Your brain, body, and mind are connected, and to realize your full potential, your limitless self, it is vital to optimize all three.

Let's Geek Out Again

Let's discuss the differences and similarities of two key neurological systems that help run the show for each of us: the Central Nervous System (CNS) and the Autonomic Nervous System (ANS).

These are two parts of your body's nervous system that are interconnected, yet they do very different things.

1. **Central Nervous System (CNS)**: This includes your brain and spinal cord. Think of it like the command center. It handles big jobs like thinking, feeling, and controlling your movements.
2. **Autonomic Nervous System (ANS)**: This part works behind the scenes, controlling things you don't have to think about, like your heartbeat, breathing, and digestion. It has two main parts: one that gets your body ready for action (like when you're stressed) and another that helps you relax and calm down afterward.

Differences:

- **Jobs**: The CNS is for thinking and moving on purpose, while the ANS handles stuff that happens 'automatically' in your body.
- **Parts**: The CNS is the brain and spinal cord; the ANS is a network of nerves going to your organs.

Similarities:

- Both parts work together to make sure your body runs smoothly, like a well-coordinated team.
- In short, the CNS is like an executive making big decisions, and the ANS is like the workers taking care of everyday tasks, both working together to keep you alive. It is critical they work in harmony.

The Vagus Nerve

Stephen W. Porges, PhD, a Distinguished Scientist at Indiana University, is the founding director of the Traumatic Stress Research Consortium. He is also a professor of psychiatry at University of North Carolina. Porges is credited with developing The Polyvagal Theory in 1995. This theory centers around the vagus nerve in our autonomic nervous system. This nerve starts at the base of the brain and connects the brain with the entire body.

Polyvagal Theory offers a novel understanding of the body's response to stress and trauma, which has significant implications for understanding addictions.

At the core of Polyvagal Theory is the concept that the vagus nerve, a key part of the parasympathetic nervous system, has two distinct branches that respond differently to stress. The older, dorsal branch can lead to shutdown or dissociative states, often seen in severe stress or trauma. The more evolved, ventral branch promotes social engagement and calming responses.

When it comes to addictions, Porges' theory provides a framework for understanding how people might use substances as a way to regulate their emotional state through the nervous system. For individuals whose nervous systems are often in the shutdown (PNS) or high-alert mode (SNS), substances like drugs or alcohol can artificially stimulate the more evolved, calming branch of the vagus nerve or numb the overwhelming sensations from the dorsal branch.

Addiction, in this light, can be seen as an attempt to self-regulate emotional states when the person is lacking healthier more effective ways to do so. Substances offer temporary relief from the extreme states of fight, flight, or freeze induced by stress or trauma. And the relief can be felt very quickly, with little effort. However, this relief is not only temporary but also maladaptive or flawed, as it doesn't resolve the underlying dysregulation of the nervous system.

Understanding addiction, and more importantly creating an effective recovery program, through the lens of the Polyvagal

Theory emphasizes the importance of developing strategies that enhance the body's natural ability to self-regulate. This perspective can lead to more holistic approaches in addiction treatment, focusing not just on the cessation of substance use (the tip of the iceberg, as discussed in Chapter 1) but more importantly, on healing the affected nervous system and rebuilding these systems for effective return to health and long-term pathway to recovery.

This is further evidence of the importance of having a Brain-First approach to any recovery program or behavior modification effort.

The Game Changer —Neuroplasticity

Neuroplasticity is the concept that can be defined as the ability of the brain and nervous system to respond to intrinsic or extrinsic stimuli by reorganizing its structure, function, and connections. In short, your brain rewires itself to change and adapt to stimuli and events in your environments. What you have today is not what you will have tomorrow—because your brain is continuously changing and adapting.

Some of you may remember in the 1980s that Nancy Reagan, First Lady of the United States, launched a massive ad campaign, that ran for years, about the effects of drug use on your brain. One of these commercials was an egg being cracked into a hot frying pan, with the message that "this (meaning the egg) is your brain on drugs," inferring that if you did use illicit drugs your brain would be 'fried'. The movement was called 'Just Say No.' This was part of the federal government's War on Drugs initiative. With good intentions, this effort had little to no positive impact on lessening addictions or providing hope for recovery. As we reflect back, we now know this campaign was misguided.

This now outdated belief was that the brain is unchangeable, and once you used substances, cells were destroyed and irreparable. Use drugs and 'kaboom', just like that, your brain was damaged, and there was nothing you could do about it – or so science and academia preached at the time.

For hundreds of years, scientists speculated that the brain changed due to the environment. In 1874, Charles Darwin studied and compared the brains of wild and domesticated rabbits. He discovered that wild rabbits' brains were significantly bigger in bulk and size than domesticated rabbits. This led Darwin to suggest his theory that a mammal's brain can and does change based on its environment and external stimuli. And it turns out that Darwin was right!

Neuroplasticity is the brain's amazing ability to change and adapt throughout life. It's like a network of roads in a city. Just as a city can build new roads or change old ones to improve traffic flow, our brain can form new connections or strengthen existing ones to learn new things or recover from emotional trauma or physical injuries.

Benefits of Neuroplasticity

The following are some of the ways we benefit from the gift of neuroplasticity

1. **Learning New Skills**: Learning something new is like constructing a new road in this network, and it can be under construction for a while. At first, this road might be rough and difficult to traverse, reflecting the initial challenge of learning. However, with repeated use and practice, the road becomes smoother and more established, making it easier to travel. This is how a skill or knowledge becomes more accessible and natural to you over time.
2. **Adapting to Changes**: Neuroplasticity also means that if an existing road (a well-established neural pathway) is blocked or damaged, say by injury or a stroke, the traffic (neural signals) can find new routes. Alternate roads can be built or strengthened to bypass the damaged area, showing the brain's ability to adapt and find new ways

to function. This is particularly important in recovery from brain injuries.

3. **Recovering from Emotional Trauma**: Just as a city rebuilds and re-routes after a natural disaster, the brain can heal and form new pathways after emotional trauma. This healing process might involve developing new coping strategies or re-framing past experiences and focusing on what you want (forward-looking) rather than focusing on the past (what you don't want) essentially laying down new roads that lead to healthier emotional responses and resilience.
4. **Recovery from Injuries**: Just as a city develops detours and new paths after a road is damaged, the brain can (depending on the injury) reorganize itself to regain lost functions even from severe physical injuries.
5. **Enhanced Cognitive Abilities**: Regular mental exercises and learning new skills can build more roads and strengthen existing ones, leading to improved memory, better problem-solving skills, and greater creativity.
6. **Emotional Resilience**: Just as a city's road network can improve to handle more traffic efficiently, the brain can develop better ways to handle stress and emotions.
7. **Aging**: A well-maintained and constantly evolving road network can keep a city functional and efficient; similarly, a brain that continues to learn and adapt can stay sharper and healthier even as you age.
8. **Recovery from Addiction**: Overcoming addiction with neuroplasticity is like redirecting traffic from a harmful, well-worn road to newer, healthier paths. Initially, the brain's pathways favor the addictive behavior, but through consistent and positive changes in habits and behaviors, new, more beneficial roads are built and reinforced. This process gradually weakens the old addictive pathways and strengthens new pathways, supporting healthier lifestyles and flourishing.

In summary, neuroplasticity is like having a dynamic and adaptable transportation network in your brain, constantly improving and evolving, allowing you to learn, recover, and maintain cognitive health throughout all stages and adversities of your life.

When it Comes to the Brain, Size Does Matter

In the 1960s a team of neuroscientists and psychologists from the University of California, Berkeley, led by Marian Diamond, PhD, and Mark Rosenzweig, PhD, discovered that a rat's brain indeed changes in size, volume and cognitive capacity based on the environment in which it lives (Rosenzweig et al., 1972).

Dr. Diamond and her colleagues found that rats living in an impoverished (lonely, without stimulation) environment had smaller brains and poor brain function, often showing signs of depression and anxiety. Conversely, when rats lived in an enriched environment (with nourishment, movement, newness, learning, and affection), much like Dr. Alexander's Rat Park which we introduced earlier in the book, their brain size was significantly larger, and their overall function and happiness had dramatically improved.

Dr. Diamond was able to confirm the concept of neurodevelopment and brain plasticity because of advances in technology.

What Dr. Diamond termed as exposure to "enriched environment" (with tunnels, wheels, social connections, exercise, fun, and loving human touch) brought about this larger brain, both in size and weight, and improved problem-solving capabilities. Conversely, an "impoverished environment" (isolated with no toys, no friends, and limited movement or play) resulted in a smaller brain both in size and weight as well as a measurable decrease in cognitive abilities to perform specific tasks.

This conclusion was ground-breaking data. Without a doubt, Dr. Diamond and her team were able to quantify that environment has a direct correlation on the anatomy and structure of the brain. As a result, the concept of neuroplasticity—the brain's ability to change, both positively and negatively—was proven true by science.

Dr. Diamond's findings were egregiously dismissed by academia and the scientific community as nonsense, in part because they were presented in the 1960s by a female scientist (very rare at the time). Science wasn't ready to hear this yet because it was mind-blowing!

In the 1990's, two significant events occurred that began to change our knowledge of the brain and the connection between brain and behavior.

First, in July 1989 President George H. W. Bush (41) signed presidential proclamation 6158 designating the 1990s to be the 'Decade of the Brain.' Over time the National Institutes of Health (NIH) would receive up to three billion dollars annually from this enthusiastic project.

Second, in May 1995 actor Christopher Reeve (Superman, 1978) was thrown from his horse while riding at an equestrian event and broke his neck. The tragic injury paralyzed him from the neck down; he used both a wheelchair and a ventilator for the rest of his life.

What emerged from this tragedy is Reeve became the (very handsome) public face for neuro-research and a catalyst trumpeting advances in neuroscience and the study of the central nervous system. His vocal support proved instrumental for both governmental bodies and the media to create heightened public awareness.

The 'Decade of the Brain' proved significant and became a launch point for science and humanity. There were many positive scientific gains that arose from the Decade of the Brain initiatives, including the following:

- Neuroplasticity—the brain's ability to rewire and restructure itself now became commonly accepted in academia, science, medicine, and with the public at large.
- Neurogenesis—the brain's ability to actually grow new neurons- was studied.
- Addictions—understanding the neural origins and connection of the brain to addiction.

- Development of new brain imaging (MRI, fMRI) and the introduction of computer-assisted neurotechnology for medical testing and direct-to-consumer options.

The Brain Goes Mainstream

We introduced Dr. Amen and his pioneering work with brain imaging, particularly using SPECT scans to help diagnose and treat mental health conditions. His work reveals how different brain areas are involved in various disorders, advancing understanding of the brain's role in mental health and addictions, guiding more targeted treatments.

Dr. Amen's 1999 book (expanded and revised in 2015), *Change Your Brain, Change Your Life* was one of the first large-scale media publications to introduce this newly accepted brain science in a manner everyone could grasp and understand.

Are We Stuck with the Brain that We Have Today?

Dr. Amen is a celebrity doctor who is a practicing psychiatrist, brain health specialist, and CEO of Amen Clinics in the US. Dr. Amen and his team use advanced neurotechnology to look at the brains of their patients first to map activity before making a diagnosis. In Chapter 2 we explained that Amen Clinics uses SPECT imaging to view and generate 3-D images of brain function.

WHICH BRAIN DO YOU WANT?

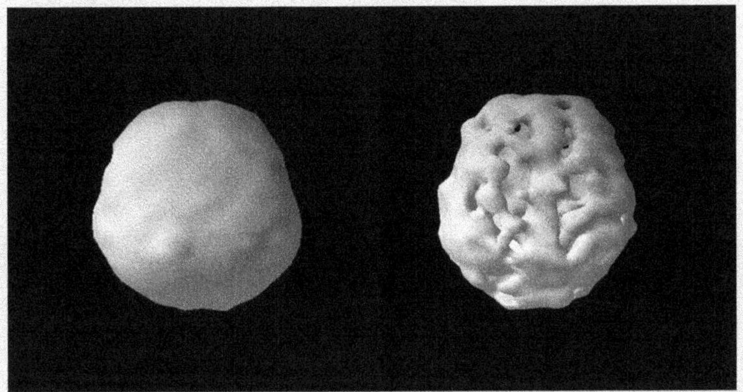

Healthy Brain SPECT Scan Alcohol Brain SPECT Scan

- The brain scan on the LEFT from the Amen Clinics SPECT imaging database shows a healthy brain with symmetrical activity throughout.
- In the brain scan on the RIGHT from the Amen Clinics SPECT imaging database, the "holes" indicate low blood flow and activity. This brain has a toxic appearance from regular alcohol consumption—just 1-2 normal-size glasses of wine per day.

For more information on the Amen Clinics Method or brain SPECT imaging, please visit the Amen Clinics website at: AmenClinics.com.

Source: Amen Clinics (AmenClinics.com)

Helping People in Recovery

Dr. Amen's pioneering work in brain imaging, particularly in the context of addiction and recovery, offers groundbreaking insights. By visually capturing the brain's activity, his methods illuminate how underlying brain dysfunction is associated with addiction and how substance abuse physically alters brain function. This imaging provides tangible evidence of these changes, making the often invisible effects of addiction visible and more understandable. Crucially, it also allows for the tailoring of treatment strategies to individual needs, enhancing the effectiveness of recovery efforts. By highlighting the brain's capacity for healing and change, his work not only demystifies addiction but also instills hope and direction in the journey toward recovery.

Change Your Brain, Change Your Life quickly became a New York Times bestseller and gained popularity through PBS TV. The title and the book itself make two key assertions. First, it is possible to change how your brain works (remember our discussions on neuroplasticity, neurogenesis, and Hebb's Law). And second, an equally powerful assertion is that if you change your brain, the trajectory and quality of your life will indeed change.

These two concepts were unheard of and ground-breaking to the general public at that time.

But there's a catch...

Much like the study done with rats by Dr. Marian Diamond, the brain can change in a positive manner or a negative manner. In turn, the outcomes in your life will mirror the change of your brain.

You can live a lifestyle that supports and helps your brain to flourish in balance or harmony to access a more optimal state. The result is that your life satisfaction will likely greatly improve, including your relationships, your wealth and prosperity, your health, your mind-body connection, your sleep, your energy, your mood, less or no need to self-medicate, no more brain fog, a sharp memory, and you gain a greater sense of autonomy.

You can also do things that will result in lowering brain function causing your brain to be out of balance. When your brain function and the nervous system are impaired or dysfunctional, you are not in an optimal state which can result in your life circumstances being more difficult with greater suffering, including:

- Health and immune problems
- Recurring financial hardships or uncertainty
- Sleep challenges (too much or too little)
- Increase in anxiety or depression (or both)
- A stronger desire to self-medicate or distract
- Relationship and career challenges
- Emotional turmoil and overall despair
- Unhappiness and loss of freedoms
- Unnecessary risk-taking
- Brain fog and memory issues

> The first time we met Dr. Amen was in 2013 at a brain conference in Vancouver, BC. After a few minutes of discussing our mutual work he invited us (Susan & Dave) to become an affiliate with the Amen Clinics, and to become Certified Brain Health Coaches. Since that time the Amen Clinics referred multiple people to our residential recovery program leading them to overcome their challenges and thrive. We've continued to stay up to date with their neuroscience based learning and enjoy a mutually beneficial relationship with like-minded professionals.

Neurocycle – Empowering Us All

Dr. Caroline Leaf, who we introduced earlier, is a renowned cognitive neuroscientist and author who has made significant contributions to the mental health and wellbeing field through her groundbreaking app called *Neurocycle*.

Dr Leaf's work has real implications for addiction and lasting recovery. She has pioneered a unique approach to empowering anyone to transformational change by leveraging neuroplasticity. Neurocycle is a 63-day structured program developed to help individuals identify and rewire toxic thought patterns, ultimately fostering mental and emotional resilience by rewiring the brain.

This trailblazing approach assists individuals in recognizing the triggers and underlying thought patterns that lead to self-destructive behaviors. By identifying the toxic thoughts and emotional responses associated with substance abuse, people in recovery gain insight into their addiction or self-defeating patterns. This awareness is essential for intrinsic lasting personal growth.

Through Neurocycle's five-step process of gathering, reflecting, writing, rechecking, and 'active reach', individuals can intentionally and progressively replace their harmful thought patterns with healthier ones. This rewiring of the brain is crucial for overcoming the cravings and impulses that often accompany addiction.

In the context of recovery, whether from addiction, trauma, or mental health challenges, Neurocycle offers a structured method to break the cycle of harmful thought patterns. This process is based on the principle that by repeatedly focusing on positive and healthy thoughts, individuals can strengthen neural pathways that support recovery and wellbeing, illustrating the brain's remarkable ability to change and adapt. Dr. Leaf's work underscores the importance of active and mindful engagement in one's thought processes as a key to effective recovery and mental health management. Over time, the new, healthier neural pathways become stronger, aiding in recovery from an addiction or self-destructive behavior by replacing the harmful thought patterns with constructive ones.

> You have the choice to live a brain-enriched or brain-impoverished life.

Dr. Leaf's work is founded on the principle of neuroplasticity giving anyone in crisis an opportunity to rewire their brain and change their life.

The ripple effect of brain-healthy lifestyle choices has a direct and significant impact on your wellbeing, performance, longevity, and your ability to flourish—or not.

Your future self is counting on you to make decisions today that result in your aging gracefully, with your mind sharp and your body strong. In doing so you will rise above it all and unlock your extraordinary.

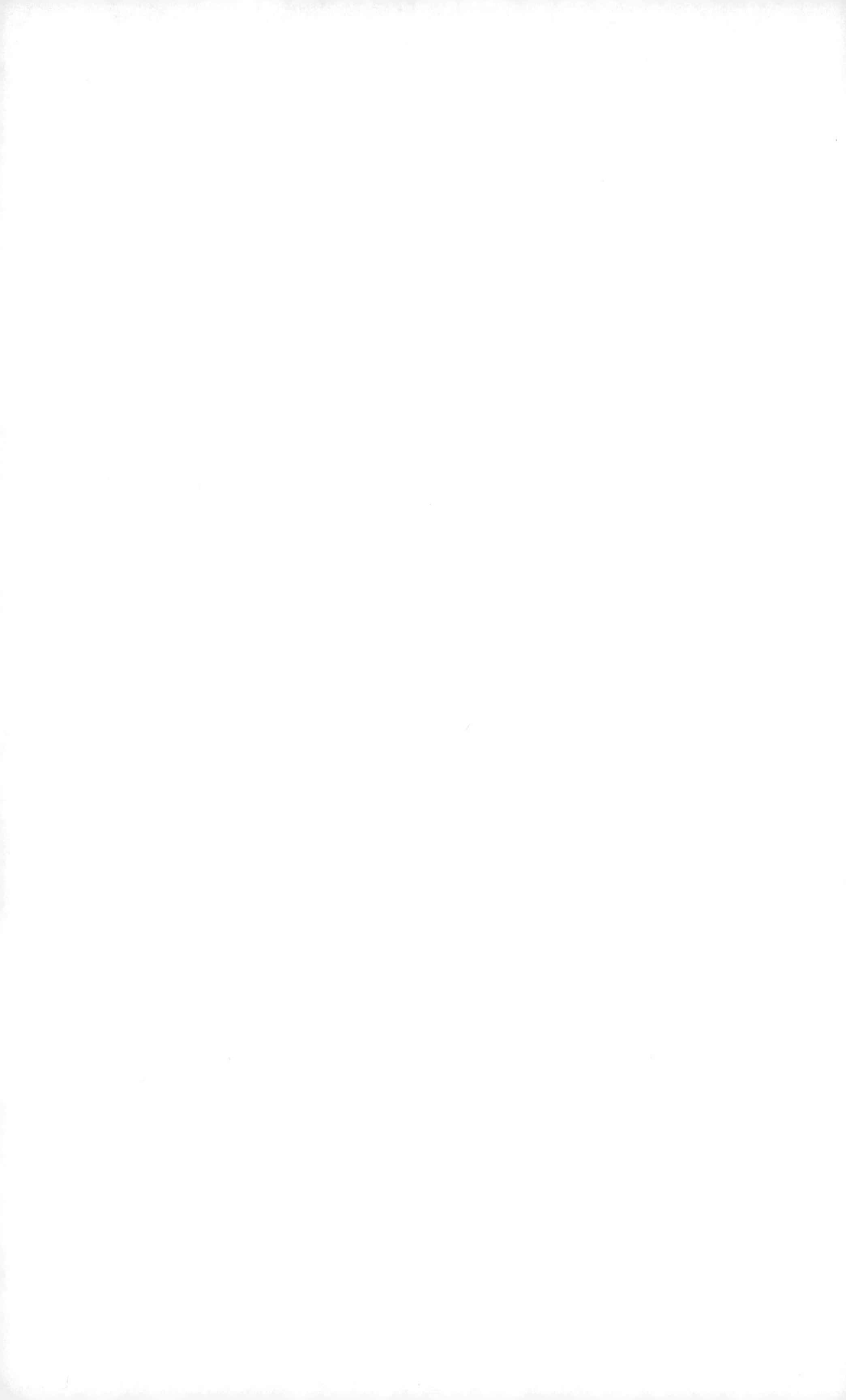

PART 2

RECOVERY BLUEPRINT

Chapter 5

Chaos to Thriving

In the midst of chaos,
there is also opportunity.
- Sun Tzu

No One-Size-Fits-All Solution

We are all unique and complex beings, and there isn't a one-size-fits-all solution to overcome human challenges. Most of the time, modern medicine diagnoses isolated symptoms without looking at the whole person.

After more than twelve years of living 24/7 with clients and coaching their families through extreme crisis, many admitting they were at their wits' end, we recognized emerging similar patterns. These patterns allowed us to develop a systematic approach guiding people to get their lives back on track. Our methodology drills down and uncovers what drives these seemingly Goliath-like challenges.

Actualized Recovery is a tailored and comprehensive solution that's easy to follow and takes people through a journey from struggle to a life that feels good.

Actualized Recovery restores physical wellbeing and freedom of mind from a range of conditions, including soft and life-threatening addiction, feeling anxious or depressed, debilitating physical health challenges, failure to launch, procrastination, perfectionism, emotional dysregulation, drifting, post-partum, eating disorders, PTSD, concussions, TBI, learning challenges, suicide ideation and more.

What are Actualized Recovery Principles?

Actualized Recovery is comprised of a set of navigating principles that are aimed at coaching and guiding individuals to achieve lasting recovery from addiction, substance abuse, self-sabotaging behaviors, physiological challenges, and life's unanticipated setbacks. These principles are based on the idea that recovery is a process of individual growth and self-actualization, and that individuals can achieve their full potential by working on themselves holistically and taking into consideration how these choices affect brain function.

Here are the key concepts of Actualized Recovery:

1. Self-Awareness: becoming aware of your thoughts, feelings, and behaviors to make positive changes in your life.
2. Self-Responsibility: accepting responsibility for your actions and behaviors, and recognizing that change comes from within.
3. Holistic Health: the importance of physical, emotional, mental, and spiritual health.
4. Meaning and Purpose: finding what matters in life beyond addiction or dependence, and working toward goals that are personally meaningful.

5. Personal Growth: a process of personal growth and transformation to achieve your full potential through ongoing self-inspired personal development.
6. Community Support: the importance of social support in achieving and maintaining goals and emphasizing the value of building a supportive community of peers and professionals.
7. Honesty and Authenticity: being honest with yourself and others, living an authentic life that matters to you and is in alignment with your personal values.
8. Mindfulness and Presence: cultivating practices of mindfulness and being present, which can help you become more aware of your (reoccurring) thoughts, feelings, and behaviors while developing a greater sense of inner peace and calm.
9. Gratitude, Appreciation, and Awe: cultivating a deliberate sense of gratitude, appreciation, and reverence for the positive and incredible aspects of your life, which can counterbalance negative emotions and experiences.
10. Resilience and Adaptability: developing resilience and adaptability (perspective) in the face of life's challenges and setbacks can help you bounce back from adversity and maintain a balanced outlook on life.
11. Service and Contribution: finding ways to give back to others (acknowledged or anonymous) and contribute to the world around you, which is essential to creating a sense of purpose and meaning.
12. Compassion and Empathy: cultivating compassion and empathy toward yourself and others, creating a foundation for kindness and connection.
13. Creativity and Self-Expression: augmenting creativity and self-expression to explore your inner mind and express yourself uniquely and genuinely.
14. Acceptance and Letting Go: learning to accept what is not within your control and letting go of attachment to outcomes or past experiences, which can help to reduce

stress and promote inner tranquility; having faith that there is a greater reason that may not be understood in the present moment.

15. Continuous Learning and Growth: the importance of ongoing learning, curiosity, and growth, both in terms of personal development and education, which can help you continue to improve your life and cultivate wisdom.

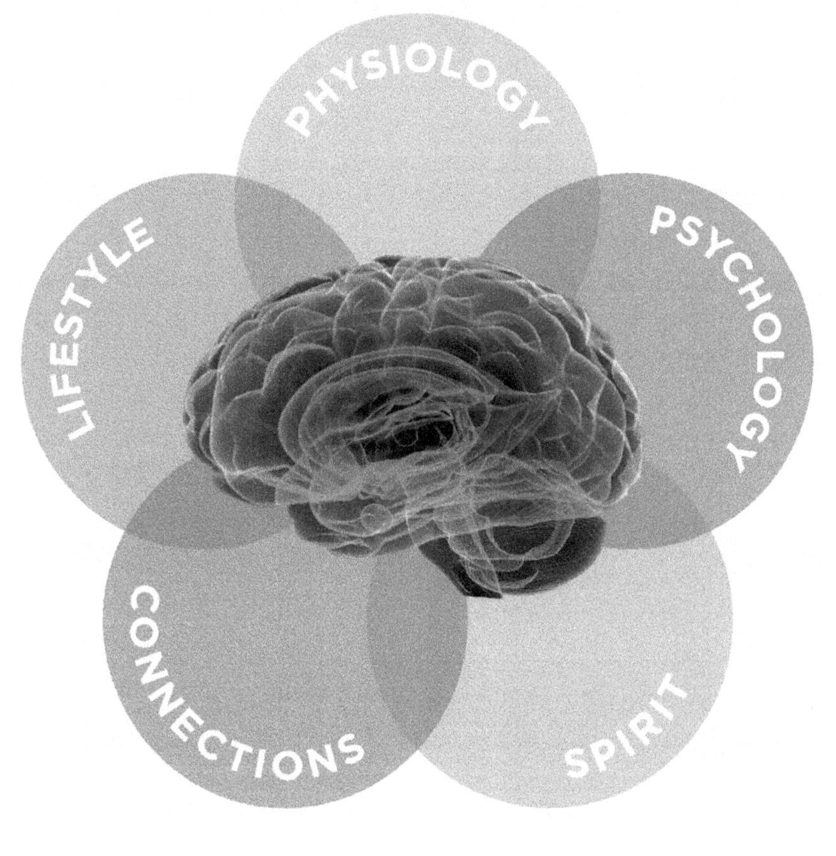
ACTUALIZED RECOVERY®
The Brain-First Approach to Lasting Recovery
PHYSIOLOGY
PSYCHOLOGY
SPIRIT
CONNECTIONS
LIFESTYLE

Integration and Balance

Finding a balance between different aspects of one's life, including work, relationships, hobbies, and self-care, and integrating these aspects into a meaningful whole life filled with abundance and freedom.

We took these 15 concepts and integrated them into five key principles that define Actualized Recovery. They are:

1. Physiology
2. Psychology
3. Spirit
4. Connections
5. Lifestyle

All five integrated principles are viewed through a brain-first lens, meaning we explore how each principle and modality will impact the brain, specifically whether it will harm or optimize brain function.

The principles of Actualized Recovery draw from a wide range of sources, including various lifestyle interventions, therapeutic modalities, spiritual traditions, and personal growth philosophies. These principles are grounded in the belief that people in recovery can achieve their full potential by accepting complete personal responsibility and working on themselves to achieve integration as a whole being.

Here's an introduction and overview of the five key principles. We have dedicated a separate chapter to each principle as they are all interconnected and equally of value to your recovery.

1. Physiology (Biology)

Maslow's Hierarchy of Human Needs was pioneered in the 1940s by Abraham Maslow, a psychologist, after studying some of the healthiest and most successful individuals of that era.

He determined the bottom tier of the pyramid of human needs is physiological. This is the foundation of human flourishing and transcendence. When basic survival needs are not met properly and consistently, your human body – including your brain – cannot function optimally. When your body is deficient, everything else in your life will likely be negatively impacted, because your primary thoughts and actions must be focused on finding and providing these physical needs.

Self-actualization
desire to become the most that one can be
Esteem
respect, self-esteem, status, recognition, strength, freedom
Love and belonging
friendship, intimacy, family, sense of connection
Safety needs
personal security, employment, resources, health, property
Physiological needs
air, water, food, shelter, sleep, clothing, reproduction

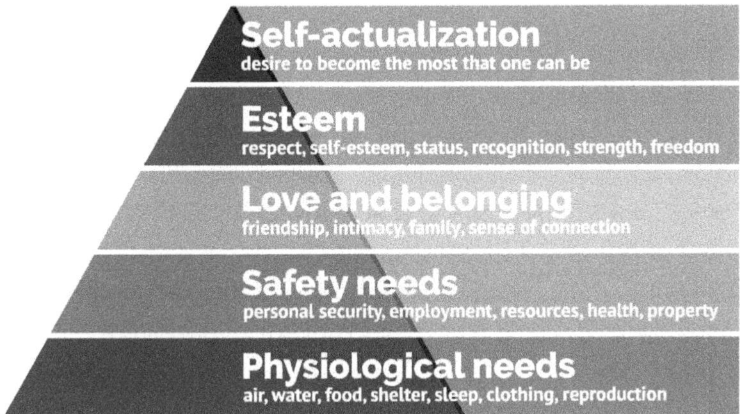

Maslow's hierarchy of needs

The basic physiological needs are air, water, nutrients through food, clothing, warmth, shelter, sleep, excretion, sex, and homeostasis. Securing these is your brain's primary motivation. Your brain determines whether these needs have been sufficiently met.

Maslow's work teaches us that it is not possible to skip this foundational step. You cannot focus on self-esteem without first focusing on and securing the basic needs. While this makes logical sense, many recovery programs and recovery efforts inadvertently skip this step or do not fully embrace the deep importance of getting the foundation dialed in. When people have been either abusing or neglecting their bodies it is omnipotent to bring every resource to this foundational step, including the resource of time.

Prioritizing physiological needs ensures a strong, resilient platform from which individuals can climb the hierarchy, step-by-step, and thrive. Understanding and fulfilling these fundamental needs is not just a starting point in recovery; it's a continuous, essential practice that supports sustained health, growth, and overall wellbeing.

2. Psychological—Mind

Change your brain and change your thoughts. In an earlier chapter, we stated that the mind and the brain are separate, but also connected and reliant upon each other. Having healthy brain function, and basic physiological needs met, creates the possibility of higher levels of creative and empowered thinking.

The foundation of the psychology that we enthusiastically endorse and teach is called Positive Psychology, which focuses on the positive events and influences in one's life, including experiences like happiness, joy, inspiration, and love, and traits like gratitude, awe, resilience, and compassion. This is a strengths-based approach to overcoming any obstacle or challenge.

Positive Psychology builds on natural character strengths and behaviors, instead of exploring deficiencies and mere survival. It keeps us fully present in the *now*, and builds a better future by leveraging the science of happiness.

The very top of Abraham Maslow's theory is self-actualization. Gone are comparisons, judgments, and making choices or acting out of a feeling of obligation which drains your energy. Becoming self-actualized is the highest level of personal psychological development, where personal potential is fully realized. This is one of the influences of why we titled our methodology *Actualized Recovery.*

3. Spirit

Developing your spiritual self in recovery is vital as it addresses a profound aspect of human experience often overlooked by purely physical or psychological approaches. Spirituality, which can encompass a sense of connection to something larger than oneself provides a deep well of strength and resilience.

Your spirit and your faith are interconnected. Your spirit is what drives you, even in times of overwhelming adversity. It's what makes you smile from the inside out. It's not about religion; faith is a part of your spirit, with the belief that your life happens for you, not to you. Your spirit defines who you are. Possessing vibrant unwavering faith, that even in the face of difficult adversity or painful setbacks, there is a greater purpose born from your spiritual self.

Gabriella Rosen Kellerman and Martin Seligman in their book *Tomorrowmind*, speak about "living a life that matters," which in turn creates long-term meaning. Determining what matters to your spirit is much easier than setting out to find what's meaningful.

Joseph Campbell (born 1904), a writer and professor of literature, outlined the steps of the Hero's Journey in a documentary film called *Finding Joe*, produced and directed by Patrick Solomon. Solomon does a phenomenal job of bringing the heros journey to life. This common story is shared in all cultures throughout time. The main character must go on an adventure into the unknown, experience battles, conflict, and hardships to emerge triumphant and transformed. It is the story that each one of us is having day to day and moment to moment. If you've done battle with addiction or dependence, know that it is part of the story that a hero will embrace as necessary. The ultimate endeavor of the hero's journey is to discover your bliss, which is a spiritual pursuit and awakening.

Abraham Maslow coined a phrase while creating the *Hierarchy of Needs* which is, "What one can be, one must be," meaning you must strive for what you are capable of and what your heart truly desires as your only pursuit; anything less will leave you yearning, despondent and lost. If you are a painter, you must paint. If you love music, you must listen to or create music. Your spirit is your intuitive guide that leads this self-actualized journey.

4. Connection—Social

Social scientists have been studying the effects of meaningful relationships and how they contribute to our lives for many decades.

In 1938, scientists began tracking the health of 268 Harvard sophomores in what was called the Harvard Grant Study. By gathering information over time, they hoped it would reveal clues to leading healthy and happy lives.

After following the surviving men (and now their families) for nearly 80 years, the world's longest study of adult life (which still continues), researchers collected a massive amount of data on the participants' physical and mental health.

In 2017, of the original Harvard cohort recruited as part of the Grant Study, only 19 were still alive. They were all in their mid-90s at the time. Among the original recruits were notables such as President John F. Kennedy. There were no women in the original study because the college was all male in 1938. However, researchers did add the wives and family members to the study over the years.

Some participants went on to become successful businessmen, doctors, and lawyers, while some ended up suffering with schizophrenia or alcoholism.

Over the years, researchers have studied the participants' health trajectories and their broader lives, including their triumphs and failures in careers and marriage. What they discovered was profound and unexpected, and not only for the researchers.

"The surprising finding is that our relationships and how happy we are in our relationships has a powerful influence on our health," said Robert Waldinger, director of the study, a psychiatrist at Massachusetts General Hospital and a professor of psychiatry at Harvard Medical School. "Taking care of your body is important, but tending to your relationships is a form of self-care too. That, I think, is the revelation."

What the study concluded is that close relationships, more than money or fame, are what keep people truly happy throughout their lives. Those ties protect people from life's discontents, help to delay mental and physical decline, and are better predictors of long and happy lives than social class, IQ, or even genes. This finding proved true (and continues) across the board for all participants in the study.

5. Lifestyle—Brain-First Healthy Lifestyle

After learning the first four principles—Physiology, Psychology, Spirit, and Connections—you can make informed choices to build environments with the lifestyle habits that will most support your recovery and ultimately embody wellbeing. This is viewed through the lens of how each decision supports or undermines optimal brain and body health, while also considering the life that matters most to you.

Lifestyle takes into deeper reflection your intrinsic values, resources (time, finance, energy), strengths, dreams, short-term targets, and legacy goals.

Your lifestyle considerations may include traditions that are important for you to honor from generations past, or establishing boundaries about what's okay and not okay for you. It's also determining what's truly important and prioritizing those things in your calendar before anything else. It includes establishing repeated routines, creating new habits that leverage the power of neuroplasticity. The way you choose to live will evolve. Being flexible - not rigid - will allow you to embrace new opportunities,

> After you put your feet on the floor in the morning, immediately say this phrase, 'It's going to be a great day.' As you say these seven words, try to feel optimistic and positive.
>
> - B.J. Fogg, PhD

new routines, and new growth while living a life of meaningful adventure.

Author, social scientist, founder, and director of the Stanford Behavior Design Lab, B.J. Fogg, PhD, wrote a compelling book called *Tiny Habits*. This book explores how making small incremental changes can have greater probability of turning into long-term habits and helping people improve their lives. We support and embrace his teachings to make small changes over time and move your momentum in the right direction. This is celebrated with each successful new action as soon as you've completed it, even if it's simply putting on your running shoes and not actually running. We will explore the brilliant findings of Professor Fogg's work in greater detail later in the book.

Lifestyle is critical to vibrant lasting recovery, as it shapes daily habits and environments that either support or undermine wellbeing. If your desire is to live a full, rewarding, and enriching life, then know that the key to longevity is your lifestyle. The best part? You are the only person who gets to vote as to how you choose to live.

The Brain-First Approach to Actualized Recovery

The brain-first approach to Actualized Recovery is a treatment approach that first emphasizes the importance of addressing neurological imbalances and disharmony in brain function that occur through trauma or stress (physical, chemical, mental, and emotional) in the physical brain.

This methodology involves a combination of neuroscientific research, brain-based therapies, and holistic lifestyle interventions to help individuals recover their wellbeing. This approach recognizes that recovery is complex, unique, and involves physiological, psychological, spiritual, social, and lifestyle factors—through the lens of what is beneficial for the brain first to achieve success in the long term.

Some of the specific elements of the brain-first approach to Actualized Recovery include:

1. Neuroscience education: Providing you with a basic understanding of how all types of trauma and stress can affect the brain, which in turn changes behavior, and how specific brain-based modalities can be used to promote recovery.
2. Neurotechnology: Using specialized equipment to reveal brain activity and provide the brain with feedback to help it correct function in a non-invasive way to bring about balance and harmony.
3. Mind-body therapies: Practices such as yoga, meditation, Qi Gong, Tai Chi, or mindfulness, provide greater awareness of your thoughts, feelings, and bodily sensations, reducing stress and promoting relaxation.
4. Experiential therapies: Creating personal awareness through tactile doing, and also experiencing modalities that engage the brain in creative solutions. By doing, there is a greater depth, engagement, and neurological growth that cannot be realized through talk therapies alone.
5. Nutrition, exercise, nature, and sleep: These lifestyle interventions promote brain health and support recovery by providing the body with the nutrients, oxygen, sunshine, biophilia, exercise, and restorative rest it needs to function optimally.

Overall, the brain-first approach to Actualized Recovery is focused on providing individuals with the specific coaching, as well as the tools and resources they need to promote healing and recovery from addiction, self-sabotaging habits, physical, mental, and emotional setbacks, and more. Recovery is achieved by addressing the underlying neurological changes that contribute to unwanted behaviors.

Our proprietary methodology is a systematic, integrative, brain-first approach to lasting recovery and sustained wellbeing that has been shown to improve with time as the brain develops and locks in advantageous patterns (new, more dominant neural connections). The reason you continue upward positive momentum is based on changing focus; when you focus on changing your brain, the brain responds in kind to continue the upward trajectory.

Using this process creates lasting positive change, a proven formula you can adapt as needed—from full-blown crisis intervention to the desire for greater vibrancy and overall quality of life.

A Beacon of Hope

Actualized Recovery marks a groundbreaking shift in addressing addiction and destructive behaviors by centering on the brain's influence over behavior. Recognizing that to change behavior, one must rewire and reprogram the brain's functioning, this approach delves into the root causes to lay a strong foundation for lasting change. It merges the latest in neuroscience with comprehensive mind-body practices and lifestyle adjustments, crafting an all-encompassing path to healing.

More than just a treatment, Actualized Recovery is a journey of transformation directed by the brain's incredible capacity for healing and adaptation. This approach uplifts individuals, offering a customized pathway of recovery that evolves with each person. It acknowledges the brain's pivotal role in driving behavior and utilizes this knowledge to foster accelerated recovery and personal growth.

Actualized Recovery shines as a symbol of hope, showcasing the human brain's remarkable resilience and offering a clear, effective route for those seeking to take back control of their lives. It is a testament to the brain's amazing ability to reprogram itself, leading you toward a life of sustained health, balance, and fulfillment. This method doesn't just address symptoms; it reorients the brain, paving the way for a brighter, more flourishing future.

Brain-First Leverages the Vast Power of the Brain

In Chapter 3, the Brain and Behavior chapter, we explained why leveraging the power of the actual physical brain is vital for sustained change. You will learn more about what you can do to correct a brain that is out of balance, and you'll discover other contributing factors for a well-functioning brain.

Let's start from the place of *it's not your fault*. You didn't set out to hurt your brain, and, in some circumstances, you had no control whatsoever for the physical, chemical, mental, or emotional trauma that occurred and created the upheaval in your life. Now though, you have the responsibility of being your own brain's advocate. Imagine it's that simple because it is! Things are either good for your brain or not good for your brain. Now ***you*** get to choose based on awareness of the facts.

Self-destructive choices, addiction patterns, and drifting in life are likely not about a moral failing or character defect. As we shared in an earlier chapter: it is not a lack of willpower, it is all about brain power. Knowing this releases shame and blame, but ***not*** accountability or responsibility.

No person *wants* to fail, be lonely, disappoint people and struggle at every turn. No 10-year-old goes to school in the morning excited to fail a math quiz, again. Everyone has greatness in them. You have greatness. And the neat thing is that greatness, or gifts, are different for all of us, and are unique to you.

Yet, people do fail. They fail the math test. They get fired from their jobs. They go into debt or bankruptcy. They get arrested for a DUI. Sometimes they repeat the same negative and destructive patterns again and again, only to hurt their family and to let themselves down, regardless of the hundreds of promises to change.

So, what happens along the way? What gets in the way of the deep desire to live with self-worth?

It's why we've written this book and why we have created a vibrant online community to support people to come together to overcome their challenges and realize a new beginning. Our community is called the **Actualized Recovery Tribe**. We meet online and have loads of support and programs. It is all based on offering hope while leveraging an integrated methodology centered around optimizing your brain with the brain-first approach to lasting recovery so you can thrive!

You can find our community at: https://www.emergoacademy.com

Navigating the path of Actualized Recovery might seem daunting, or you might question its effectiveness for you. Rest assured, these concerns are common.

Based on extensive feedback and grounded in the latest research, years of experience, and the program's impressive success rate, here are some suppotive responses to common hesitations:

Hesitation 1: It seems like a lot of effort.

- The lifestyle you're currently living is most likely already demanding. Actualized Recovery replaces uncertainty with clarity. Experiencing pride in your achievements will lead to a newfound self-appreciation, something that's hard to imagine now, but becomes a reality in an actualized life.

Hesitation 2: What if it doesn't work for me?

- Neuroplasticity works for everyone! Success hinges on your brain to change positively. You'll learn a customized, integrative approach, requiring decisions that best suit you within established guidelines. Actualized Recovery incorporates diverse human thriving strategies, offering ideas that will resonate and ignite a spark within you, prompting action because they align personally with your values.

Hesitation 3: What about the fear of change and the unknown?

- Stepping out of your comfort zone can be both intimidating and exhilarating. It often leads to heightened expectations as others witness your transition from dependency to independence.

Hesitation 4: Fear of Failure

- Failure is a part of growth. Actualized Recovery provides tools and support to help you overcome setbacks, focusing on long-term success and resilience. The intention is not perfection; it is growth.

Hesitation 5: Concerns about Social Isolation

- Recovery may change your social landscape, but it also opens opportunities to new, supportive relationships and communities that align with your healthier lifestyle.

Hesitation 6: Doubts about Self-Worth

- The program focuses on your strengths, helping you rebuild self-esteem and recognize your worth, reinforcing that you deserve happiness.

Hesitation 7: Financial and Time Commitment

- Investing money and energy into recovery is a commitment to upgrade your future. Frankly, you are worth it! There are no shortcuts, but with consistent action, change happens quicker than you think.

Hesitation 8: Lack of Immediate Results

- Recovery is a journey. Our program emphasizes gradual, sustainable progress, teaching diligence or grit, and celebrating small victories along the way. It's also good to remember it may have taken years, or even decades to get you to this *aha* point in your life. Be kind to yourself and focus only on doing your best because that's all any of us can truly do.

You are not alone. Most of your concerns or worries may feel unique to you, but rest assured, everyone has these doubts. Remember this is about embracing a brighter future. Each step brings you closer to the life you want to live.

The Adventure from Victim to Hero

Transitioning from a victim to a hero, especially in the context of overcoming addiction, is a transformative process that shifts the narrative from dependency and blame to autonomy and responsibility. In the victim mindset, individuals often find themselves trapped in a cycle of blaming others, justifying their actions, or complaining about circumstances. They rely on external rescuers, be it other people, substances, or situations, to dictate their life's direction. This dependency creates a sense of powerlessness, where life happens to them, rather than being the changemaker.

However, embracing the role of a hero marks the beginning of a compelling personal comeback story. A hero on their journey acknowledges their own wisdom in shaping their life. They move away from blaming external factors, and instead take ownership of their actions and choices. This shift is crucial in addiction recovery. It involves recognizing that while you cannot control every aspect of life, you do have the autonomy and strength to make positive decisions and changes.

It's about writing a new story where challenges are met with courage. In this narrative, every step forward is a testament to your independence and determination to create a life free from the shackles of addiction.

This shift from victimhood to heroism is not just about overcoming addiction; it's about redefining yourself and rediscovering your strengths, passions, and capabilities. It's a path that leads to a life of deep joy, freedom, and autonomy.

Bookending Your Days

There are two powerful times of the day to set new positive habits in motion: when you wake up, and before you go to sleep. These are the *bookends* of your day.

Hal Elrod's *Miracle Morning* concept is a powerful tool, particularly for those on a recovery voyage, blending a structured start to each day with meaningful practices. This routine includes moments of silence (like meditation or prayer), positive affirmations, visualization of goals, physical exercise, engaging in reading, and reflective writing or journaling. Each element plays a vital role in shaping your mindset for the day ahead.

For someone in recovery, this method is more than just a daily routine; it's a lifeline. The practice of meditation provides a calm start, allowing for mental clarity and introspection, essential for overcoming challenges. Affirmations and visualization act as daily reminders of personal strengths and aspirations, focusing on what you want. Physical exercise not only boosts health, but also improves mood and resilience, essential in the journey of recovery. Reading broadens perspectives and encourages continuous learning, while journaling offers a space for self-expression and tracking progress.

Establishing these habits in the morning creates a balanced framework, instilling discipline and a sense of purpose. Consistency is key in maintaining recovery, as it nurtures positive habits that support a healthier lifestyle. The *Miracle Morning* effectively rewires the brain, fostering new, beneficial neural pathways that make positive behaviors more natural and sustainable.

The *Miracle Morning* isn't just a set of activities; it's a transformative routine that provides stability.

We encourage you to start each day with a mindful practice of gratitude. When you wake up, while still nestled in your bed, take a moment to reflect on three things you're thankful for, and more importantly, delve into why these things matter to you. This focus on the *why* activates your emotions, which is a crucial aspect of truly experiencing gratitude. Engaging in this practice stimulates your conscious awareness and accelerates positive neural changes in your brain.

To make this a habit, consider using a visual reminder, like a sticky note on your bedside lamp or bathroom mirror. This note can be the first thing you see when you wake up, serving as a prompt for your gratitude practice.

Similarly, before you drift off to sleep, keep a journal on your pillow, and take a few minutes to jot down three positive aspects of your day. Reflect on why these moments were meaningful. Committing to this nightly ritual for at least four weeks can lead to measurable changes in your neural pathways. Many who have adopted this practice report feeling more serene at night. They find that negative thoughts, which might have previously dominated their bedtime, disappear. Consistent practice has shown to result in better sleep quality, and a sense of rejuvenation and optimism upon waking.

Incorporating these gratitude practices at both ends of your day complements the *Miracle Morning* routine, reinforcing a mindset of positivity and thankfulness that can fast-track your recovery.

The integrated, holistic approach of Actualized Recovery ensures a more thorough, personalized, and sustainable path to healing, emphasizing the synergy between the brain and all facets of life for true, lasting recovery and expansion.

So, in the spirit of curiosity and growth let's *cannon-ball* into the deep end, and explore the five integrated principles of Actualized Recovery.

Chapter 6

Physiology
The First Principle

...you have the power to change your brain.
All you have to do is lace up your running shoes.

- John Ratey, MD, Harvard University

Physiology First

How would you care for your vehicle if you were gifted one car for your entire lifetime and could not trade it in for a new one?

You've been gifted one dynamic body and mind designed to last you for a lifetime. Your one irreplaceable brain is responsible for the quality of your relationships, learning, memory, emotions, intelligence, wealth, career, resilience, and how well your body operates. It's your responsibility to treat your brain and body with the utmost respect, and we are going to provide you with an updated owner's manual!

The Growth of Neurological Conditions

We say this a lot – physiology drives psychology, meaning if your body isn't healthy then your mind is at increased significant risk of being unhealthy. We are a mind-body integrated system.

Neurological symptoms are on the rise like never before. Symptoms like neuropathy, brain fog, migraines, anxiety, depression, addictions, Lyme's, vertigo, MS, Parkinson's, tinnitus, tics, focus and concentration, head pain, neck pain, back pain, mysterious joint pain; these are all brain and nervous system conditions.

This may come as a complete shock to you. One of the major drivers to the alarming rise in these conditions comes from the nervous system not getting the fuel that it requires for high energy output. To support the nervous system to overcome these disruptions, it needs uninterrupted glucose sugars from a natural source. Your nervous system is made up of nerve cells and these cells all exist on sugar. The vagus nerve needs sugar to exist. More details regarding your critical need for glucose later in this chapter.

Somewhere around seventy thousand years ago, the brains of our ancestors—the sapiens—underwent profound alterations, including enlargement and rounding of the parietal and cerebellar regions of the brain. These regions contribute to planning, long-term memory, language, tool use, and self-awareness. The newly complex intelligence of homo sapiens allowed us to respond to environmental challenges in exponentially smarter, faster ways. Nothing on earth has been the same since (Kellerman and Seligman 2023, 19).

> "Use it or lose It."
> - Marian Diamond, PhD

Human Physiological Needs

To nurture their newly upgraded brain, our ancestors needed to make caring for this new version a priority. The good news is that with the greater intelligence it was easier to know and remember what to do to survive.

Physiological needs refer to things that are necessary for survival, such as breathable air, food, water, sleep, and warmth. *Safety* needs provide you with the consistent ability to meet physiological needs (like having healthcare and knowing your water is clean), and to be physically safe (like adequate shelter or being in a large group).

In the US, 6 in 10 adults have a preventable chronic disease, and 4 in 10 adults in the US have two or more preventable chronic diseases. The leading causes of death and disability, and leading drivers of the nation's $1.4 trillion spent in annual healthcare costs, are key lifestyle risks for chronic disease according to the Centers for Disease Control and Prevention (CDC). These lifestyle risks include tobacco use, poor nutrition, lack of physical activity, and excessive alcohol use.

> I had to find the interconnection of my brain together with my physiology.
>
> - Wim Hof

We were surprised to discover that most people we have worked with (since 2011) had many of these same lifestyle risks. Clients who were struggling:

- had been drinking little to no water daily
- rarely ate anything that contained nutrients to nourish their brains
- did not prioritize sleep
- were very shallow breathers
- had moderate to severe digestion complaints
- did not move their bodies regularly, or would put their bodies at risk by pushing themselves too hard.

This was consistent for teens, young adults, and adults.

We spoke in Chapter 5 about Maslow's Hierarchy of Human Needs. What's important to acknowledge is that these are human physiological **needs**, not a *want* or merely a *desire*.

Resetting Your Brain

In our residential program, Week One was the Restoration Phase. Each person's journey of recovery begins with developing consistency with hydration, nourishment, movement, and establishing daily routines based on natural circadian rhythm. Creating routines based on your evolutionary clock is supportive of your wellbeing because your internal 24-hour clock regulates physical, mental, and behavioral processes.

Resetting and rejuvenating your brain, and building physiological strength and resilience, is the kickoff to thriving. You can't bypass it. It's essential for the foundation of your successfulness now, and for your future self.

In this chapter we are going to focus on some of your physical needs from your brain's point-of-view. No matter your current starting point, your brain and body are resilient and can improve very quickly.

Creating a vibrant healthy brain will ripple into every part of your being. When your body and brain are functioning optimally, your resources of time, money, and energy can be used to create the life of freedom that you truly want.

In this modern era, people are in constant threat of being exposed to pathogens, toxins, viruses, chemicals, and heavy metals. These can embed within the brain and wreak havoc with behaviors. Luckily, humans are designed to be able to detoxify these neurotoxins.

As you age, while following a brain-first approach you won't likely need to stress and worry about what diseases you may end up with. Instead, you're setting yourself up for the best possible way to age gracefully. You get to continue to do what brings you bliss and focus on the legacy you want to leave behind.

Having a healthy brain and body will naturally increase your wealth, because you will have more resources, including energy, to devote time to what brings you prosperity.

We have a medical system that is incredible at *crisis care*. There have been astounding advancements in lifesaving surgeries and stabilizing critical care patients. What has ***not*** advanced at the same pace is care for people struggling with chronic health problems, mental health challenges, or substance use issues.

Your brain health is your number one responsibility if you want to achieve your full potential.

What we heard in our recovery program was a similar story from hundreds of people. They were feeling low and/or anxious. Sleep was elusive. Some were coping with troubles by self-medicating for relief. Others were having dark thoughts or had even attempted to end their lives. Seeking help and solutions, they went to a doctor, psychiatrist, other allopathic or holistic health professionals, or hospital emergency. Then they typically walked out with one (or more) diagnosis, recommendations, maybe prescriptions, or a referral to a specialist who gave them more of the same advice, but no real answers about the cause.

We asked each client if any of the attending medical professionals had ever asked them what was going on in their lives; what they were eating or drinking; how their evening routine was set up to encourage sleep; how much time they were using technology; how much they were in nature; how much physical exercise they did; how demanding was their level of stress at work, home, or school; if they had meaningful relationships, or if they were lonely. The answer was always 100% "No!"

Beyond Symptoms: Addressing the Cause with Lifestyle Interventions

You can't correct a neurological condition or imbalance with medicine or a medication. You can assuage symptoms for short-term relief (hopefully). But seeking relief from symptoms is a short-lived reprieve at best. Theses treatments don't delve into the root cause of the imbalances we experience. This is why medications for neurological or cognitive issues are taken repeatedly.

Lifestyle interventions are transformative practices that guide your brain and body toward a balanced state, called homeostasis. By integrating these lifestyle changes into your daily routine, you unlock the opportunity to relish each day with ease and grace and to reap the rewards of exceptional performance that positively impact every aspect of your life. These lifestyle interventions include:

- sleep
- hydration
- whole, living foods (not ultra-processed)
- nature (biophilia)
- movement
- breath
- play, fun, laughter, hobbies
- learning and curiosity
- connections with friends, family, and community
- mindset

The absence of medicine isn't the cause of health issues; often, it's the lifestyle choices we make. By focusing on these fundamental lifestyle opportunities, you hold the key to not just feeling better but unlocking your extraordinary.

As neuropsychiatrist Dr. Amen points out, psychiatrists typically do not look at the organ they are attempting to treat. This is the only medical specialty to base their diagnosis on symptom clusters, as self-reported by the patient.

According to the American Psychiatric Association (APA), for people struggling with Substance Use Disorder (SUD) or an addiction, *"People with a substance use disorder may have distorted thinking and behaviors. Changes in the brain's structure and function are what cause people to have intense cravings, changes in personality, abnormal movements, and other behaviors. Brain imaging studies show changes in the areas of the brain that relate to judgment, decision making, learning, memory, and behavioral control."* (source: https://www.psychiatry.org/patients-families/addiction-substance-use-disorders/what-is-a-substance-use-disorder)

The APA confirms that SUD is a brain structure and brain function issue, ***not*** a brain chemistry issue.

National Institute on Drug Abuse (NIDA) basically agrees with the APA. NIDA has thirteen principles for treating drug addiction. The first principle states: *"Addiction is a complex, but treatable, disease that affects brain function and behavior."* (Source: *Principles of Drug Addiction Treatment: A Research-Based Guide*).

If the problem, then, is connected to brain structure and brain function, wouldn't that mean the solution can be found in balancing or optimizing brain structure and brain function?

The following excerpt is from the jacket of a book called *Saving Normal: An Insider's revolt against out-of-control psychiatric diagnosis, DSM-5, big pharma, and the medicalization of ordinary life,* written by Allen Frances, MD. Dr. Frances is professor emeritus and former chair of the Department of Psychiatry and Behavioral Science at Duke University School of Medicine, and Chair of the DSM-IV Task Force. DSM is the Diagnostic and Statistics Manual, which is the *bible* of psychiatry. Frances states, *"Anyone living a full, rich life experiences ups and downs, stresses, disappointments, sorrows, and setbacks. These challenges are a normal part of being human, and they should not be treated as psychiatric disease...we also shift responsibility for our mental well-being away from our own naturally resilient and self-healing brains."*

Frances felt compelled to write *Saving Normal* when the most recent DSM-5 was introduced in 2013 (updated as DSM-5-TR released in 2022). It included huge leaps in pathologizing normal human behavior.

In his eye-opening book, Frances calmly states, "Prescription drug abuse has become a bigger problem than illicit drug abuse" (Frances 2013, 95). Prescription drug abuse impacts every corner of our world with catastrophic effects. We have certainly all seen this with the devastation of the opioid crisis.

Can We Change a Brain?

This is the very first question that we the authors of Actualized Recovery asked, which began an unexpected adventure that continues today.

Marian Diamond, PhD (whom we have referenced previously) was one of the first to break through the old paradigm of believing that the brain could not change if it was impacted by trauma or toxins including alcohol or drugs. Dr. Diamond was born in 1926. Given she was a woman and was born when she was, she became a neuroscientist against great odds. We can all celebrate her tenacity. Dr. Diamond was the first female graduate student in the Department of Anatomy at the University of California, Berkley, and is considered one of the founders in the field of neuroscience. She dedicated her life to passionately studying the brain.

In 1966, Dr. Diamond led a team that discovered neuroplasticity, the brain's ability to change and grow larger while living in an enriched environment (we will define what an *enriched environment* is soon). This discovery is fundamental to our work and being able to achieve incredible long-term results with people recovering from various challenges.

Dr. Diamond also discovered that when living within and enduring an impoverished environment (the opposite of an enriched environment), the brain shrinks in size and functionality. The team studied the impact on rats living under these poor conditions and found they were low functioning, struggled with tasks, and suffered from depression and anxiety (among many other challenges). With a lack of nutrients, stimulation, and comfort, their brains became measurably smaller.

When rats lived in an enriched environment, their brain increased in size. They lived longer and happier lives. Essentially, these rats thrived!

Despite being rejected for more than two decades, neuroscience eventually recognized Dr. Diamond's findings on neuroplasticity. This is one of the greatest breakthroughs in the study of the brain.

A human's brain is constantly restructuring and reorganizing how it functions, essentially how it's wired, by responding and adapting to life experiences. This impacts a person's behavior (either positively or negatively) and the expressions of feelings. This exciting finding provides a tremendous opportunity to help those who feel challenged to be able to optimize their life.

Dr. Diamond discovered five things that foster an enriched environment to help focus and create your best brain:

1. Diet
2. Exercise
3. Challenge
4. Newness
5. Love

We will now spend some time on these first two discoveries that defined an enriched life for Dr. Diamond's rats. We'll explore the other three in the next chapter on Spirit.

Hydration and the Brain

Imagine a large, juicy, ripe grape. This is your happy, hydrated brain. Now imagine a small, shriveled raisin. This is your sad, toxic, dehydrated brain. It doesn't take a neuroscientist to figure out which brain will function better!

Not having enough fluid can negatively impact your brain function and behavior in several ways:

1. Dehydration: When the body is dehydrated, the brain can shrink in volume and pull away from the skull, which can cause headaches and impair cognitive function. Even mild dehydration can impair cognitive function, including memory, attention, and reaction time.
2. Fatigue: Dehydration can cause fatigue and lethargy, which can impair mental alertness and cognitive function.
3. Impaired mood: Dehydration can negatively affect mood, leading to irritability, anxiety, and depression.
4. Impaired decision-making: Dehydration can impair decision-making and judgment, making it more challenging to think clearly and make sound decisions.
5. Memory impairment: Dehydration can impair memory and recall, making it more difficult to retain and retrieve information.

6. Reduced cognitive flexibility: Dehydration can reduce cognitive flexibility, making it harder to adapt to new situations and switch between tasks.
7. Toxic load: Being dehydrated keeps toxins within your cells because hydration is the vehicle by which toxic substances (that cause havoc) can be eliminated from your body.

Overall, not providing your cells with enough water, fresh fruit and vegetables, coconut water (clear), and living water within uncooked fruits and raw vegetables, can have a significant negative impact on brain function and behavior. Therefore, it is essential to stay adequately hydrated to maintain optimal brain function and autonomous behavior. Upgrade your brain by quenching your thirst and expect better physiological robustness and mental acuity as well as many other facets of your life to improve.

Ultra-Processed Food IS a Rising Substance Addiction

We are massive fans of Dr. Chris van Tulleken's research and lectures. He has authored the book, *Ultra-Processed PEOPLE: The Science Behind Food That Isn't Food.*

Chapter 7 of this book is titled, *Why it isn't about sugar...* Chapter 9 is titled *...or about willpower.*

Sugar has been *canceled* because it's been wrongly accused of causing harm.

In a culture where *nutritional experts* are selling science that has been funded by parties for their gain (following the money), we have become sicker, slower, and stupider. Why? Because blaming one food and favoring another is not the solution; we need to widen the lens and ask different questions.

In the mid-1970s, obesity became prevalent for the first time in our human history – across all ages, genders, and other demographics. Could this be because suddenly more people than ever before were lacking in willpower and failure of personal moral responsibility in all of the different global communities? Seems unlikely, doesn't it?

So, what changed? Ultra-processed foods became part of the mainstream household diet, that's what. Food manufacturers had finally convinced women that these convenience foods were nutritionally superior. They also influenced women by launching campaigns that suggested they deserved to get out of the kitchen and live with more freedom. It was brilliant.

The advertising to integrate processed foods into the American diet was incredibly clever. In the 1950s, General Mills (the makers of Wheaties and Cheerios) invented a persona who they named Betty Crocker, and she was the perfect woman! They launched robust radio and magazine exposure with ads that brought the modern kitchen to life and were endearing to women.

Almost every home had copies of the Betty Crocker Cookbook, which was designed to teach women how to cook for their families using ultra-processed ingredients with as much confidence as they had when cooking with recipes that had been passed down through the generations. Then they even created a Betty Crocker cookbook for kids.

In 1965, General Mills unveiled the Pillsbury Doughboy, who became an iconic figure. They brought to life an adorable, animated giggly character to sell the new line of Pillsbury's refrigerated dough products (biscuits, dinner rolls, sweet rolls, and cookies). In commercials and magazine ads Poppin Fresh, aka the Pillsbury Doughboy, showed the public how easy it was to make fresh breads and treats. People went wild to purchase these – never questioning the quality of the ingredients.

By the mid-70s, everyone was indoctrinated. The plan worked. In only one generation, our whole food system changed. But the requirements of our physical bodies did not.

The human body is a beautifully synchronized system that can take nutrients from the (real) foods that we eat, and through a well-choreographed and highly evolved digestive system, use this nourishment for cellular growth, maintenance, and the fuel that energizes us.

Processed food is different from ultra-processed. Grinding, cutting, cooking, mashing, extracting, fermenting, smoking, salting, and curing foods have been practiced for hundreds of thousands of years. The processing of food has shaped our physiology by utilizing the benefits of making foods taste good, last longer, and be easier to work with. This is a way of eating that uses foods that were or are alive to create our meals.

Ultra-processing is different.

Rice, corn, soy, and wheat (broken down into fats, protein, and carbohydrates) are the base cheap commodity crops that you'll find in ultra-processed foods. They are then typically mixed with commodity oils – palm, sunflower, canola, mixed vegetable oils, and then mixed with protein isolates.

Left in this state, these ingredients would taste and look horrible, so additives to emulsify, stabilize, preserve, flavor, and color, must be added to enhance texture, visual appearance, and taste. Once completed, these 'foods' have a nearly infinite shelf life and cost very little...but they have been stripped of all nutrition during the ultra-processing.

In the UK and Europe, there are roughly 2500 food additives and these are somewhat regulated. In the US, there are between 5000 – 15,000 food additives – there is no 'list' and the Food and Drug Administration (FDA), the entity that is expected to regulate these additives does not have a list of everything that manufacturers of ultra-processed foods use.

Real food can't compete with ultra-processed foods that have been designed in a lab to hack into your brain's joy response.

A research group led by Carlos Monteiro, who is an MD and Senior Nutritional Professor in Brazil, defines that part of the purpose of ultra-processed food (UPF) is profitability, being easily marketed and easy to sell.

Analysis of 281 studies from 36 countries found that ultra-processed food addiction was estimated to occur in 14% of adults and 12% of children. These statistics were published by researchers in the British Journal of Medicine.

Now, researchers say the way some people consume such foods could meet the criteria for diagnosis of substance use disorder.

Behaviors that meet these criteria include intense cravings, symptoms of withdrawal, less control over intake, and continued use despite such consequences as obesity, binge eating disorder, poorer physical and mental health, and lower quality of life, they said.

The researchers, from the US, Brazil, and Spain, said: "Refined carbohydrates or fats evoke similar levels of extracellular dopamine in the brain striatum to those seen with addictive substances such as nicotine and alcohol.

"Based on these behavioral and biological parallels, foods that deliver high levels of refined carbohydrates or added fats are a strong candidate for an addictive substance."
https://www.theguardian.com/science/2023/oct/10/addiction-to-ultra-processed-food-affects-14-of-adults-global-study-shows

Brain Food—How Sweet It Is

Firstly, Susan wants to make clear that for most of her adult life, she followed a paleo and keto-type eating plan. Her training as a sports nutritionist in the early 2000s was all about consuming enough protein and fats. In her early adult years, she tried the Atkins and South Beach diets – which the current keto trend has recycled. Susan, like many aging people, was feeling the physiological, mental, and emotional effects of a diet that encourages high fat and low carb. Over time (the time frame depends on the person's exposure to toxins and pathogens) these fat and protein diets result in physical and mind fatigue, and require the person to get energy from other stimulants to survive, because as stated earlier, every cell in your brain and body requires glucose for energy. When Susan learned that the key to vibrant energy was all about focusing on clean carbohydrates, it came as the biggest revelation. Initially, she had a very hard time accepting this new information. As Dave and Susan and their clients transitioned to eating more fresh fruits, freshly juiced fruit and green juices, smoothies without fat or protein, fresh leafy greens, vegetables, and starchy vegetables like potatoes, sweet potatoes, and squashes – the transformation was incredible and played an undeniable role in rejuvenating the brain and body.

The brain requires a constant supply of glucose (energy) to carry out its essential high-energy demands such as thinking, intellectualizing, analyzing, remembering, and controlling body functions. Glucose is the primary and essential source of energy for the brain because it is the most efficient fuel that can be metabolized quickly and easily by the brain cells.

While fat and protein can be used for energy, they are not as efficient as glucose. For instance, fat molecules are too large and complex to be quickly broken down and metabolized by the brain cells. Protein molecules are mainly used for building and repairing tissues in the body, rather than for energy production.

Furthermore, the brain is dependent on a continuous supply of glucose as it cannot store large amounts of this energy. When glucose levels in the brain are depleted (due to low sugar ingestion and/or high stress), the brain cells can become damaged, leading to cognitive impairment, seizures, and even coma.

"The brain is dependent on sugar as its main fuel," says Vera Novak, MD, PhD, an HMS associate professor of medicine at Beth Israel Deaconess Medical Center. "It cannot be without it."

The Harvard Medical School published an article in 2016 stating, *"Glucose, a form of sugar, is the primary source of energy for every cell in the body. Because the brain is so rich in nerve cells, or neurons, it is the most energy-demanding organ, using one-half of all the sugar energy in the body. Brain functions such as thinking, memory, and learning are closely linked to glucose levels and how efficiently the brain uses this fuel source. If there isn't enough glucose in the brain, for example, neurotransmitters, the brain's chemical messengers, are not produced and communication between neurons breaks down. In addition, hypoglycemia, a common complication of diabetes caused by low glucose levels in the blood, can lead to loss of energy for brain function and is linked to poor attention and cognitive function."* (source: https://hms.harvard.edu/news-events/publications-archive/brain/sugar-brain).

The National Institute of Health (NIH) published an article titled, *'Increased Intake of Vegetables and Fruits Improves Cognitive Function among Chinese Oldest Old: 10-Year Follow-Up Study',*

May 2023. They concluded that adults who frequently consume fruits and vegetables maintained higher levels of cognitive function. They concluded, *'Encouragingly, there exists a positive correlation between psychological well-being and cognitive function among older adults'* who regularly consumed both fruits and vegetables. (source: https://www.ncbi.nlm.nih.gov/pmc/articles/PMC10180819/).

The Journal of Nutrition published an article, *'Intake of Vegetables and Fruits Through Young Adulthood Is Associated with Better Cognitive Function in Midlife in the US General Population,'* (August 2019). The authors concluded that eating a diet with whole vegetables and fruits rich in fiber is attributed to better cognitive performance and supports healthy aging. (source: https://www.sciencedirect.com/science/article/pii/S0022316622166903)

Low Carb – Low Cognitive Function

"A High Fat High Protein Diet Makes You Sick, Slow, and Stupid..." That was the title of Susan's presentation to a group of women entrepreneurs. At the end of the presentation, a majority of these women connected with Susan to learn more – because each of them had the symptoms of low physical energy and mental stress and were noticing cognitive decline. All of the women Susan spoke with were following a low carbohydrate, high fat, and higher protein style of eating.

Every week, there seems to be a new way for us to eat that is THE best diet. Knowing what is best can seem very confusing. We hope to clarify nutrition *from a brain point of view* to feed the organ that drives the quality of physical and mental health and vibrant longevity of your life.

As we stated earlier in the book, you have around 100 billion neurons in your brain and trillions of cells in your body. ***Each one requires glucose to function.*** The trend today is to brainwash everyone to think that the brain is made primarily of fat and, therefore, needs fat to function. This is a huge myth. We are told that sugars hurt the brain. We are told that no-sugar or low-or-no-carb diets are the solution to health. This misinformation could be one of the root causes of many addictions and behavioral challenges for many people.

Conventional science knows that the brain runs on sugar. Medical textbooks teach that without sugar, even for a short period of time, our brains are in peril.

To be clear, your brain's primary fuel source is glucose.

A healthy brain is mainly made of glycogen (stored energy food source) and low levels of fat. You don't want a fatty brain any more than a fatty liver.

Being starved of glucose can result in the brain shrinking. We shared earlier that brain size *does* matter. And you definitely want to have the biggest brain in the room!

Your brain's electrical energy—and how it communicates and functions—runs on high-quality sugar. Having excess fat in your brain impedes the processing speed of its internal communication.

Toxic heavy metals in the brain, such as mercury, copper, aluminum, lead, and cadmium, also impair the brain's communication signals, resulting in addictive behaviors and mental health and cognitive challenges. These metals can lodge in the brain beginning in childhood from medications, pollution, ultra-processed foods, body products, and many more sources. However, heavy metals in our neurons are a very important topic for another time. The relieving news is that a diet focused on critical and necessary carbohydrates can support your brain in flushing metals and other accumulated toxins out of your brain cells.

A glucose deficiency can occur when someone embarks on a restrictive, no-sugar or low-carb diet. Over time, the essential glycogen (energy) that your body has stored in your liver and brain becomes depleted from the high fat and protein consumed. This outcome is the same regardless of the source—plant ***or*** animal. The liver is the first organ to lose its valuable storage; your brain gets robbed next.

The result is that you will likely crave substances or develop adrenaline-seeking behaviors because the brain is searching for energy, and these things temporarily boost the fatigue brought about by the lack of glucose. The brain perceives that alcohol is one of these sources, but because it is processed, it does not provide the brain with what it truly requires. Alcohol is a fake source of glucose that wreaks destruction on the brain and liver, not to mention your life.

The sugar your brain needs and thrives on comes from natural sources, is unrefined, and is blended with other critical components, such as trace minerals, trace mineral salts, phytochemical compounds, antioxidants, anthocyanins, vitamins, and other nutrients.

Sugars that are not good for the body include alcohol, candy, conventional baking, sodas, and prepackaged (high corn syrup) foods. Your body longs for the natural sugars in fresh fruits and starchy vegetables. The healing glucose supports neurotransmitters and counters cravings and addictions by calming and soothing your brain.

Glucose Deficiency occurs when glucose is depleted within cells of the body and brain. Your wellbeing depends on eating all types of fruits and starchy vegetables like potatoes, sweet potatoes, squash, and even raw honey. Every cell in the human body runs on glucose as the primary fuel. Your brain needs critical glucose levels to function well and make good choices. If you are deprived of glucose, you will become obsessed with getting it because your brain knows that your survival depends on it.

Insulin Resistance occurs when there is too much fat from a high-fat, high-protein (another form of fat) diet. The more fat in the blood, the more insulin is needed to force the sugar through the fat saturation to enter the sugar-starved cells. This is true with plant-based diets and animal diets. This is a massive problem for your cognitive health. Dementia is now commonly referred to as *Type 3 Diabetes*.

Adrenaline Surge Dependency is when you are addicted to the feeling of the coming *high*. Being depleted in glucose sets you up for another life-smashing setback, known as *adrenaline addiction* or *adrenaline surge dependence*. When glucose isn't available, your adrenal glands pump adrenaline into the body so that you can function. Think of adrenaline as the backup generator when the power goes out. This adrenaline *rush* becomes addictive. Adrenaline compensates for the lack of glucose (natural sugar). Excessive adrenaline is corrosive and creates physiological distress and serious health conditions. Adrenal fatigue is one of the unintended effects of a low-carbohydrate (fruits and starchy vegetables diminished) diet, or a way of eating that heaps fat on your essential carbs, making it nearly impossible for your cells to extract the precious glucose.

When you're addicted to adrenaline, you get hooked on the *adrenaline high* feeling, and you yearn and obsess for substances like caffeine, buzz (energy) drinks, chocolate, or other sugary treats and snacks. Even certain behaviors can give you that adrenaline buzz you crave, including anger, raging, aggressive fast driving, gambling, extreme sports, bungee jumping, cliff diving, or other risk-taking behaviors. Anything that gives you the energized rush.

Being addicted to adrenaline isn't sustainable long-term; the brain gets confused, brain fog sets in, and you feel fatigued and drained. What's actually needed to offset these symptoms are glucose and trace mineral salts for the brain to energize in the form or fruits, leafy greens, and vegetables, preferably loading up on these precious life-sustaining sugars early in the day (grab an apple when you go out the door!), without adding fats or proteins.

Factors that play a part in adrenaline dependence include frequent life stressors, uncertainty, immense pressure (real or self-imposed), and emotional and/or physical abuse. Even lack of sleep or poor sleep hygiene can cause your body and brain to be sluggish, so you crave a *jolt* of something to get through your morning.

Being human is hard. We face heartbreak, betrayal, fear, struggle, confrontation, chaos, and shock – sometimes all in one day. In times of stress, distress, and emotional and physical upheaval, we need even greater sources of glucose to combat the surging adrenaline that is released to provide energy to deal with a stressful situation. If you don't have glucose stored, your cells will crave glucose for survival. You know this is true. When you're under stress, you crave sugar, and your brain craves carbohydrates.

> What I aim to do here is to deliver in plain English the inspiring science connecting exercise and the brain and to demonstrate how it plays out in the lives of real people. I want to cement the idea that exercise has a profound impact on cognitive abilities and mental health. It is simply one of the best treatments we have for most psychiatric problems.
>
> - John J. Ratey, MD

Before the end of this chapter, we will talk about what you can do to help your brain and liver replenish the stored glycogen.

In 2008, best-selling author and renowned psychiatrist John Ratey, MD, published a pivotal book called SPARK. This wonderful read embarks upon a fascinating and entertaining journey through the mind-body connection. It presents startling research proving that exercise is truly the best defense against everything from depression to ADD, addiction, aggression, menopause, and even Alzheimer's. His book is filled with amazing case studies correlating exercise and benefits for the brain. So much so, it became one of our core curricula for our recovery program.

Here is a short YouTube video titled "Exercise And The Brain', from the book *SPARK* by Dr. Ratey https://youtu.be/OPhcft_hwV8

Where You Can Begin

Below are some actions you can take to bring to life what we've discussed in this chapter:

- Begin the day with 16 (or more) ounces of clean drinking water with freshly squeezed lemon. This supports the body in eliminating toxins accumulated overnight. Aim to drink half of your body weight (pounds) in ounces of water each day. Example: If you weigh 180 pounds, you'll want to drink 90 ounces every day of water, or clear coconut water. Fresh juices (no pulp) are incredible for hydration. Fresh, uncooked fruits and vegetables contain *living water*, which can be even more hydrating than liquids because of the vitamins and minerals that give your digestion something to hold onto as it processes.

- Add brain and liver-healing glucose and carbohydrate sources like fruit, raw honey, squash, potatoes, and other root vegetables to your diet, away from fat/ protein. Make friends with healthy carbs and fruit, curtail your fat and protein intake, and reclaim the healthy life you are meant to live!
- Make your sleep sacred. Create evening routines that follow a natural circadian rhythm. This includes sleeping 7-9 hours a night and maintaining it consistently 7 days a week.
- Dr. Matthew Walker, PhD, is a professor of neuroscience and psychology at the University of California, Berkley, and also the founder and director of the school's Center for Human Sleep Science. Dr. Walker has deeply studied how sleep affects the brain and body. He has published the book *Why We Sleep* (2017), and we highly recommend this, as well as his TED Talk and podcast, to learn how sleep affects your brain (and much more). Dr. Walker is brilliant at breaking down why sleep in all stages is necessary and how you can craft your environment to achieve iconic sleep.

Chapter 7

Psychology
The Second Principle

The secret of change is to focus all of your energy not on fighting the old, but on building the new.

- Socrates

Psychology—Your Mind is the Software

Psychology is the scientific study of the human mind and behavior. It seeks to enhance our understanding of human nature and improve the wellbeing of individuals and society as a whole.

> The mind is the force that drives neuroplasticity. This is why I say the mind changes the brain.
>
> - Dr. Caroline Leaf

Defining the Mind

Neuroscientist, Dr. Caroline Leaf, states:

> "The mind and brain are actually two very different, but interconnected, entities. As a neuroscientist, this reality is the foundation of my life's research and work: The mind works through the brain but is separate from the brain. The mind uses the brain, and the brain responds to the mind. The mind also changes the brain. People choose their actions—their brains do not force them to do anything. Yes, there would be no conscious experience without the brain, but experience cannot be reduced to the brain's actions."

Let's take a closer look at the difference between your brain and your mind. Your physical brain is constantly changing. Every moment—with each new experience—your brain is learning and adapting at a physical level. Your mind is how you actually ***experience*** life. Your mind is responsible for how you think, feel, and choose, which is unique to you. The physical brain, in contrast, is responding at a physiological level to the mind's interpretation of every conscious (awake) and unconscious (asleep) experience.

Your mind is always listening, learning, and rewiring your brain. Always. If you say, "I'm powerless," your neurons create that reality based on your command.

Human brains are incredibly complex. When stimulated by the mind, the brain's structure changes because thoughts are rewiring and building new brain structures. ***The mind and brain are separate but rely on each other to function.*** It is exactly like our analogy that your brain is the hardware, and your mind is the software that brings the computer to life.

The brain is an intricate neuroplastic responder. This essentially means that each time your mind activates your brain, it responds in various ways, including neurochemical, genetic (yes, you can influence your genes), and electromagnetic changes. This, in turn, grows and changes infrastructures in the brain that build or wire new physical thoughts.

Brain waves are the brain's response to what a person is thinking, feeling, and choosing. The data is visual evidence, which can be measured through technology to show that the mind is functioning, that the mind is working, and that one is, in fact, alive.

The energy that is measurable within the structure of the brain is the thoughts that create structural changes within the brain. These changes are neuroplasticity in action from thinking, feeling, choosing, and doing.

The good news is you can learn how to manage your mind. You have the power to make feelings of depression, stress, anger, and anxiety work ***for*** you instead of against you. Imagine being able to bring balance back into your brain and life. That is precisely what you can do. When you have autonomy over your thoughts, unwanted behaviors are within your control.

Logotherapy

Logotherapy, developed by Viktor Frankl, is a type of psychotherapy that focuses on helping individuals find meaning and purpose in their lives.

> Between stimulus and response there is a space. In that space is our power to choose our response. In our response lies our growth and our freedom.
> - Viktor Frankl

Frankl believed that the primary motivation in human beings is to search for meaning, and by discovering that meaning, we can overcome challenges and achieve psychological wellbeing.

As a young Jewish psychiatrist in Austria, Frankl was beginning to develop his theory while working in a psychiatric hospital with female suicidal patients. In 1942, he was taken by the Nazis and sent to a concentration camp. His father, mother, and wife died in the camps while Viktor observed the brutality and degradation around him. He ascertained that those inmates who had some meaning in their lives were more likely to survive.

One of the core tenets of logotherapy is the idea that a gap exists between any stimulus (an event or situation) and our response. In this gap, we have the freedom to choose how we will respond to the stimulus. Frankl's famous quote best captures this idea: "Between stimulus and response, there is a space. In that space is our power to choose our response. In our response lies our growth and our freedom."

This concept suggests that while we may not have control over certain events or circumstances that happen to us, we do have control over how we interpret and react to them. Even in the face of adversity or suffering, we can choose our attitude and find meaning in our experiences. This ability to choose our response empowers us to transform challenges into personal growth and development opportunities. This is the place of freedom.

When it comes to addiction recovery, logotherapy can be especially relevant and impactful. Addiction often stems from a lack of meaning and purpose in life, leading people to seek solace in substances or behaviors. By applying logotherapy principles, those in recovery can explore the underlying factors contributing to their addiction and find new meaning to live.

For instance, someone recovering from substance abuse may face triggers or difficult situations. Instead of resorting to drugs, alcohol, or behaviors, logotherapy encourages them to recognize the gap between the stimulus and their response. By choosing a healthier and purposeful response, such as seeking professional support, pursuing hobbies, or being of service to others, they can strengthen their resilience and influence their recovery.

Logotherapy's focus on finding meaning in life aligns with the belief that everyone has the ability to create a purposeful and fulfilling existence, even in the face of addiction challenges. It emphasizes personal responsibility and encourages individuals to take charge of their mental and emotional wellbeing, essential elements in overcoming adversity.

Logotherapy is a powerful psychotherapy approach, emphasizing the importance of finding meaning and choosing the responses to life's events. Its application to addiction recovery allows individuals to address the root causes of reliance and develop healthier coping strategies. By recognizing the freedom to choose how they respond to stimuli, those in recovery can cultivate a more purposeful and fulfilling life journey, breaking free from the enslavement of addiction and embracing newfound meaning. They are rewriting their story and thereby rewiring their brain.

Intrinsic versus Extrinsic | Inside Out versus Outside In

Sustainable change occurs in the brain when a person implements an inside-out approach. What does this mean? It's like the difference between telling someone that they should change, or the person themselves realizing that there are benefits to making changes. The mind and brain adapt better to new ideas and patterns when invited to change organically, not when forced.

The therapeutic modalities we have witnessed that create the most powerful mind shifts are the ones that we will focus on in this chapter. They encourage the development of new positive neural networks intrinsically, in other words, from the inside out. These therapies create new habits because they create awareness of past behaviors and current circumstances by engaging all of the senses, with the sole purpose of overcoming past traumas and troubles by seeing yourself as the changemaker. Once again, Hebb's Law comes into action: the neurons that fire together, wire together, and become stronger than old self-destructive neuropathways.

> People do not resist change. People resist being changed.

Some of the ideas we share in this chapter are the ones our clients experienced the most release from. However, they are only a fraction of the therapies available to support the growth of mind and functional brain change.

Positive Psychology

Positive psychology is an evidence-based approach to studying human thought, feelings, and behavior, focusing on strengths instead of deficiencies. It's centered around building experiences that focus on the good in life instead of trying to repair the bad. This is a huge departure from historical (or classical) psychology. Its purpose is to increase people's lives from ordinary or average to *great* by exploring and imagining positive experiences. It successfully shifts perspective from the limited view of examining past negative life experiences.

The most commonly accepted definition for the field of positive psychology is: *"*Positive psychology is the scientific study of what makes life most worth living*"* *(Peterson C., 2008).*

The revolutionary field of positive psychology contemplates a broad range of topics, including character strengths, optimism, life satisfaction, happiness, wellbeing, gratitude, awe, compassion, self-compassion, self-esteem, self-confidence, hope, self-actualization, and rising above.

Discovering Virtues and Character Strengths

Ryan Niemiec and Robert McGrath are two of the leading figures in the positive psychology movement and, more specifically, within the organization called the VIA Institute on Character. VIA stands for *Virtues in Action.*

The VIA (Values in Action) Strengths framework is a cornerstone of positive psychology that identifies and leverages individual strengths and virtues. Developed by psychologists Martin Seligman and Christopher Peterson, this approach diverges from traditional psychology's emphasis on fixing weaknesses. Instead, it catalogs 24 character strengths grouped under six broad virtues. These strengths are considered universal across cultures. Knowing and living your strengths is a game-changer in human performance and recovery. Focusing on and intentionally living your gifts, the things that make you unique, in a positive way, rather than solely addressing your flaws, brings greater hope, builds resilience, and allows us to shine.

A person struggling with an addiction will typically beat themselves up and emotionally criticize themselves more than anyone can possibly know. Often, they see themselves as a failure or weak.

When you understand your gifts and focus on your unique character traits, building a career and life that is in harmony with your strengths, you create a tapestry of hope and are better able to rise above any addiction.

Emphasizing your virtues matters because it shifts focus from what's wrong to what's strong.

Here's the link to the take the free character strengths quiz for yourself: https://www.viacharacter.org/

Experiential Therapies

Experiential therapies for recovery are therapeutic approaches that focus on engaging individuals in hands-on, interactive experiences to facilitate emotional healing, personal growth, and recovery from various psychological and emotional challenges. These therapies often involve activities that encourage self-exploration, expression, and processing of emotions in a safe, supportive, and perhaps even fun environment. Experiential therapies can be particularly effective for individuals who struggle to express themselves through talk therapy. Some examples of these are: Play Therapy, Art Therapy, Equine-Assisted Therapy, Music Therapy, Psychodrama (acting out real-life scenarios or role-playing), Adventure Therapy (hiking or rock climbing to build resilience, and promote problem-solving skills), Dance/Movement Therapy – great for self-expression and improved body awareness – Wilderness Therapy, Drama Therapy, and many more.

We have utilized all of the above experiential therapies and others over the years. A profound realization can occur when all the senses are engaged, and people forget what they are *supposed* to be saying and doing.

Play Therapy

Dr. Stuart Brown wrote a book called *Play: How it Shapes the Brain, Opens the Imagination, and Invigorates the Soul*. Through extensive research, Dr. Brown has proven that play is anything but trivial. In fact, he proved quite the opposite. Play is filled with purpose and is a biological drive as integral to our health as sleep or nutrition. ***We are designed by nature to flourish through play.***

Play supports our mental health, improves our ability to relate to others, and increases our drive and hope for the future. When play is missing or inadequate, it can have negative consequences in these areas (and many more). Instead, taking time to play will give you a more optimistic outlook and mitigate stress levels during challenging life events.

Trust, flexibility, optimism, problem-solving, emotional regulation, perseverance, openness, and belonging are all enhanced when our lives are play-filled. That's worth reading again!

The daily schedules of clients in our recovery program would include individual and group play with board games, badminton, swimming, basketball, pickle-ball (a crowd favorite), building snowmen and snow forts, mountain coasters, ropes course, geocaching, escape rooms, rock climbing, golf, and even axe throwing. Many of the teens and adults (and sometimes their families) who we worked with initially scoffed that frivolous play could make any difference in their serious negative thought patterns.

They very quickly learned the tremendous power of fun and laughter. As the old adage goes, laughter is the best medicine.

The first year we opened, we didn't have a budget to purchase games. One of our coaches invented the sock toss game, where we used laundry hampers and rolled-up socks. Each team got to toss their socks from the second level to the main level to score. We still remember the cheers and encouragement from teammates, the camaraderie, the friendly competition, and the inevitable squeals of laughter that could be heard in every corner of the property!

It was during these activities that we witnessed the spark of life returning.

Magically, depression washed away. Anxiety disappeared. The emotional pain and scars vanished. Everyone was in the moment, focusing on the game and fun. Later, in reflection, this was used as a tool to help people understand the power of being mindful and remaining in the moment, focusing only on what you can control.

Art Therapy

"Creativity in and of itself is important for remaining healthy, remaining connected to yourself and connected to the world," states Christianne Strang. Strang is a professor of neuroscience at the University of Alabama Birmingham, and the former president of the American Art Therapy Association.

This philosophy extends to any type of visual creative expression: drawing, painting, collaging, sculpting clay, writing poetry, cake decorating, knitting, scrapbooking, whatever it is that ignites your inner artist. The sky's the limit!

"Anything that engages your creative mind—the ability to make connections between unrelated things and imagine new ways to communicate—is good for you," shares Girija Kaimal. Dr. Kaimal is a Drexel University professor and an art therapy researcher. She leads art sessions with members of the military suffering from traumatic brain injury and caregivers of cancer patients.

Practicing art and tapping into your creative flow allows the walls that have seemingly been built around your mind—from trauma, depression, anxiety, grief, or addiction—to dissolve.

Most people in our program nervously shared that they were not artistic, not very creative, and would do just about anything to try and get out of doing art, much less make themselves vulnerable by sharing it with others.

One accomplished therapist on our team was gifted at helping clients become comfortable within minutes. One strategy was to initiate the session by playing a game she called, 'scribble tag.' It worked like a charm to bring about laughter and ease the transition into the *vulnerable* art project. These included tracing the outline of their own bodies on a large sheet of paper and using the power of art to draw or paint to express how they were really feeling inside their bodies.

Another was to build a mask using their own faces to make the mold. They would paint the exterior of the mask to reflect the persona they shared with the world. The inner side of the mask was how they felt when they weren't hiding behind that outer mask. The two sides of the mask were always profoundly different. When the person explained the differences, it was like they were building a bridge that closed the gap from fake to real. This proved time and time again to be a powerfully revealing and very therapeutic *art* project.

Clay was another tactile medium that offered clients deep personal insights. Using clay to form something they no longer wanted in their lives, they then used the same clay to create something they did want.

These classes were always astonishing. Literally, what could not be shared with words was brought to the surface with art. Most people were stunned (in a good way) with their own creation. What's more, it was incredible to witness the emotions that were released given the opportunity to explain the personal meaning of their creation. The dark clouds parting to let the light in. This is the intrinsic change that we referred to at the beginning of this chapter.

It is a *rising up* that occurs from unexpected processing of past sometimes unconscious memories. It occurs in a way that the mind can process a past experience and make sense of the feelings. When this occurs change can happen in an instant.

This would be a good time to share that we spent a lot of money on tissues! There were several boxes in each room, especially during therapeutic art sessions. Witnessing the healing and transformation was profound.

Equine Therapy

Horses have a strong, natural desire to be of service and interact with people, as the following article explains (https://www.washingtonpost.com/creativegroup/zoetis/how-horses-help-humans-heal-and-thrive/).

There is a magic that is simply inexplicable when people have experiential interactions with horses. They are born teachers and natural healers, having the ability to see past the facade of how humans present themselves to the world. They can intuitively and effortlessly connect with the most authentic self.

Equine therapy provides profound and, in many cases, permanent shifts, promoting human transformation and personal growth. It all transpires through the wisdom of the horse. This heart-centered approach of putting to rest the pain of the past helps people develop a deep inner connection with the non-judgmental horses and themselves.

Horses have a unique way of tapping into people's core emotions. Horses sense energy. They have a knowing that supersedes what a person may be comfortable sharing verbally.

In one very profound session—and there were many—a young woman was in the ring with a beautiful and powerful mare. The young woman had been quiet since arriving a couple of weeks earlier. After the facilitator worked with her on building a heart-centered connection and taught her how to set clear boundaries, the horse sensed exactly what the young woman needed her to do.

The woman stood still as the horse slowly walked around her. The horse quietly stood behind the woman and leaned its head against the young woman's back. Gently and slowly breathing. They stood as one. Tears started flowing freely.

The woman's hurt and pain from years of struggle began releasing at that very moment. They stood together with neither one moving for another 15 minutes, the horse seemingly absorbing and releasing from her what had been bottled up deep inside.

From that day on, there was a different energy from this young woman. There was a lightness and playfulness that continued to emerge.

Cognitive Behavioral Therapy (CBT)

Thoughts ⟹ Feeling ⟹ Action (Behavior)

Cognitive Behavioral Therapy (CBT) is a type of psychotherapeutic treatment. It helps people learn how to identify and change destructive or disturbing thought patterns that negatively influence their emotions and behavior.

CBT combines cognitive therapy with behavior therapy by identifying maladaptive thinking patterns, emotional responses, or behaviors and replacing them with more beneficial patterns.

The focus is based on creating awareness of automatic negative thoughts and then changing them. It is these automatic negative thoughts that can contribute to and worsen emotional difficulties, depression, and anxiety, which begin the spiraling-down patterns that can land us in a dark place. These spontaneous negative thoughts also have a detrimental influence on mood.

The brain generates and processes an average of 70,000 - 80,000 thoughts each day. The challenging part is that 95% of these thoughts are the same things that we've been regularly thinking about each day.

Thoughts create structures and patterns of neural networks within the brain's structure. One is destined to live out the same day without challenging these recurring thoughts. People become stuck in what's called neuro-rigidity. Phrased another way, this is automatic negative thoughts.

CBT can be a powerful modality. Yet for many, it is seemingly impossible to change these negative thought patterns, even though people are greatly motivated to change. People are desperate to live a better life yet lack the willpower to sustain the momentum of new thoughts.

Why?

For many people who have become entrenched in discordant thinking habits, the physical brain itself has sustained change that doesn't allow CBT to *stick*.

Brain-First Cognitive Behavioural Therapy

BRAIN ⟹ Thoughts ⟹ Feeling ⟹ Action (Behavior)

Working initially to restore the brain's physical balance and harmony—which we spoke about in detail in the previous chapters—one gains the flexibility of the structural brain to release the stuckness that occurs when the brain has sustained physical, chemical, mental, or emotional traumas and distress.

By supporting the organ itself (brain) to relax and regulate energy flow, people can let go of negative thought patterns much more easily and without resistance, making CBT far more efficacious.

Automatic Negative Thoughts—ANT Stomping

In his pioneering book, *Change Your Brain, Change Your Life,* Dr. Amen does a beautiful job of identifying nine types of negative thoughts that commonly infiltrate people's minds.

They are labeled as ANTs, which stand for Automatic Negative Thoughts. "Negative thoughts invade your mind like ants at a picnic," according to Dr. Amen. These nine different negative thoughts are ways your thoughts lie to you and make situations seem worse than they actually are. One way to view these nine descriptions is like nine different species of ants.

An easy exercise is identifying the type of ANT you may resonate with. This simple action can release the power these thoughts can have over you.

How to Exterminate Your ANTs!

1. Examine your thoughts and notice an ANT. Acknowledge it, write it down if possible, and then talk back to it. Challenge the ANT in order to interrupt the downward spiral.
2. When you hear yourself say an ANT, immediately stop and correct the statement with the truth.
3. Read the common ANTs below and use the following process to kill the ANTs.

Here are the nine categories Dr. Amen has identified:

1. *All or nothing* thinking is black or white thinking that everything is all good or all bad. Here's an example: You've gone for a walk every day for four weeks, and so you now think that you are the most disciplined person on the planet. Then one day you miss your walk. You feel like your thoughts are beating you up. As a result, you now think you're lazy and lack drive. You then use this pattern as an excuse to become a couch potato.

Recommendation: Be kind to yourself and acknowledge that life happens. Get back on track and celebrate your effort!

2. *Always* thinking, meaning your words over-generalize. It includes statements like, "I will never be able to stop eating junk food."

Recommendation: Acknowledge that you have absolute control over what you choose.

3. Focusing on the negative. This ANT allows you only to see the negative, like "I know I lost 10 pounds, but I wanted to lose 15, so I'm a failure."

Recommendation: Reframe and focus on the win. Acknowledge that you're well on your way toward your goal and create a new plan.

4. Thinking with your feelings. This involves instilling a negative statement with a feeling. For example, "I feel like I'm trapped in this job that I hate, and there's no way out." Feelings can lie and make the situation seem overwhelming and hopeless.

Recommendation: Write down one way that your job provides you with freedom. Brainstorm about ways you could add to your skillset that could open up more opportunities.

5. *Guilt beating* is defined as words like 'should,' 'must,' 'have to,' which all involve excessive guilt to control a behavior. Another way to define this is known as *self-shaming*.

Recommendation: No one resists change itself; rather, people resist being forced to change. Using guilt or shame as a motivator can work, but it can also come with other unwanted feelings. Instead, what could be an encouraging statement that excites you to change?

6. *Labeling* is calling yourself or someone else degrading terms. In this case, you are using the ANT labeling. It is saying or thinking statements like "I'm a loser," "I'm a failure," or "I'm so lazy." This way of thinking provides you with the excuse never to start.

Recommendation: Whenever you say, "I am," follow it with a powerful statement that builds faith in your ability.

These last three are the most poisonous ANTS!

7. *Fortune-telling* is defined as predicting the worst possible outcome. It is catastrophizing everything. Example: "I found a strange lump, and I'm sure it's cancer."

Recommendation: Know there are things that happen, which need attention and clear thinking. Stay level-headed in a place of reality and use your clever mind to look at options that will provide clarity.

8. *Mind-reading* is when you think you know what someone else is thinking without proof because they haven't told you and you haven't asked questions. Example: "I just know that my boss hated my presentation."

Recommendation: Ask curious, open-ended questions to seek clarity and truth.

9. *Blame.* Of all ANTs, this is the most sabotaging. This is when you blame others (people, government, media, etc.), or circumstances (weather, traffic, establishments, etc.). This is when you take no responsibility for your problems and failures. This toxic thinking keeps you stuck in a victim mindset. Example: "I know I missed work, but it's not my fault the alarm did not go off when I set it."

Recommendation: Take responsibility and ownership for how you react to adversity.

**Source: Dr. Amen and Amen Clinics*

Writing a New Story

> I am not what happened to me, I am what I choose to become.
>
> - Carl Jung

With each thought that you have, you're writing a story in your brain. Then, you're choosing to believe that story. Rewrite your story to be positive, and then believe that one.

Here's a song by the Canadian band, USS, titled *Big Life (26 Letters)*. This is an inspiring song that may lead you to write your new story: https://www.youtube.com/watch?v=UDcTNYHQU14&t=10s

Here is an excerpt of the lyrics:

I learned to not hold on so tightly
'Cause letting go seems to go so well
Fearlessness is the key to the castle
Make your own heaven, make your own hell

You don't know how powerful you are
Rewrite your history
It starts with

Twenty-six letters
Stitch them all together
Make a big life, a big life
Infinite to nothing
From zero back to something
Make a big life, a big life
A big life, a big life

Everyone loves a comeback story...so write your next chapter and 'Make a Big Life.'

Chapter 8

Spirit
The Third Principle

The human spirit is more powerful than any drug –
and that's what needs to be nourished:
with work, play, friendship, family.
These are the things that matter.

- Robin Williams (1951 – 2014)

Spirit is often seen as the source of life, wisdom, and morality and is believed to be the source of emotions, thoughts, and feelings.

When you recognize your spirit, your vibrational energy is one of love, kindness, compassion, unity, community, and harmony. Spirit shines when there is sincerity and integrity in your words and actions.

Everyone needs to know—at the level of your being—you matter. You need to know that what you do matters. You need to know that your life matters.

Spirit is not righteous, superior, or shaming. Your spirit is the opposite of narcissism. It's not radical. Spirit builds bridges rather than tears them down.

The human spirit is constantly drawing you toward your greatness and highest self, which is collaborative and caring. Spiritual growth is about internal up-leveling of the self and not wanting to change others. It's being passionate about caring for the environment and rights of all humans, while committing to being part of the solution. It is not about evoking blame or needing recognition for beliefs.

Spirit can be seen as a multifaceted concept encompassing many different meanings and interpretations. It can be understood as a divine or supernatural entity, an essential aspect of human nature, or an intangible force that imbues living beings and things with vitality, meaning, and purpose.

In a philosophical context, spirit can refer to the essential nature or character of something. For example, the spirit of a community or organization might refer to the collective values, beliefs, and attitudes that define its identity and direction.

Francesc Torralba once said, "Spiritual intelligence is not a religious consciousness."

Your Spirit and Your Brain

George Vaillant is a psychiatrist and Harvard professor who, for 35 years, led Harvard's 70+ year Study of Adult Development. In this study, he followed participants from teenagers as they grew into great-grandparents!

Spiritual Evolution, by George Vaillant, explores the relationship between spirituality and human development. He draws on research from a variety of fields, including neuroscience. This research delivers evidence that spiritual experiences are an essential part of our human memories and play a significant role in personal growth and wellbeing.

Vaillant proposes that spirituality is an innate human quality that has evolved over time and is rooted in the brain's biology.

For example, Vaillant highlights the work of neuroscientist Andrew Newberg. Dr. Newberg used brain imaging technology to study the brains of individuals engaging in spiritual practices. Dr. Newberg's research has shown that certain areas of the brain become more active during meditation or prayer, indicating that these practices have a neurological basis.

His research found that spiritual practices help us to navigate life's challenges to determine meaning and purpose, and result in positive psychological outcomes such as resilience, altruism, and creativity.

George Vaillant emphasizes the importance of a holistic approach to spirituality, which integrates personal experience *and* cultural traditions. He discovered that spiritual growth is an ongoing process that requires both inner exploration and engagement with the wider world. This insight ties in to the topic of our next chapter, which is about connection.

His book discusses research showing that individuals who engage in regular spiritual practices, such as meditation or prayer, tend to have lower levels of stress and better overall health outcomes. Vaillant recognized that these practices help individuals cultivate a sense of inner calm and resilience that help them cope with life's challenges.

Vaillant shares: *"The human capacity for positive emotions is what makes us spiritual...to focus on the positive emotions is the best and safest route to spirituality that we are likely to find."*

Below is an overview of the seven key positive emotions as presented in Vaillant's work:

1. **Faith** – Vaillant makes the distinction between belief and trust. Belief is a set of thoughts. It's cognition. Faith, on the other hand, refers to the *emotion* of trust. Trust is defined as the world having meaning and that love, and kindness exist.

2. **Love** – All mammals are programmed to love. Human beings are ***the*** most wired to experience love. Hence, love is the shortest definition of spirituality.

3. **Hope** - Hope is all about believing your future will be better than your present. Later in this book, we're going to talk about just how powerful hope is when related to recovery.

4. **Joy** - Although joy is the least researched of the primary human emotions, it's also one of the most powerful. Feeling joy involves the brain's limbic system (emotional brain area for memory and motivation), including the amygdala, ventral striatum, and prefrontal cortex.

5. **Forgiveness** - Forgiveness requires the capacities for empathy and for future-thinking. Paradoxically, it benefits the one who is doing the forgiving even more than the one forgiven. That means it doesn't serve you to continue stewing on the self-poisonous resentment. Without practicing forgiveness, this toxic way of thinking keeps you stuck in your negative thought patterns.

6. **Compassion** - Vaillant tells us that love and compassion are very different. Love is about connecting with someone we find appealing, but compassion is the desire to separate someone (even if we don't see them appealing) from their suffering.

7. **Awe** - Awe and a sense of the sacred are perhaps the most *spiritual* of the positive emotions. It's that sense of connection to something bigger than yourself, in which you connect to the whole of humanity.

In another powerful read, Dr. Dacher Keltner shares the new neuroscience of how awe can transform your life in his book, appropriately named, *Awe*.

Overall, the effects of awe on brain function and activity provide further evidence of the importance of awe for human flourishing. By promoting positive emotions, reducing anxiety and fear, improving physical health outcomes, and increasing social connectedness and empathy, awe can have a range of incredible benefits for brain health and cognitive function.

Contemplative practices that can lead to more awe-someness in your brain include:

- Music
- Reading
- Walks in the woods, referred to as *forest bathing*
- Meditation
- Mindfulness
- Play
- Watching children play
- Dance
- Art
- Simply *being*

For many, this sense of the sacred and contemplation is found within nature. We mentioned nature biophilia in Chapter 6, referring to the human attraction to and feeling connected with nature. Here are profound findings about spirit and nature: 81% of Americans believe in spirit. Half of those people say that they find it in nature.

Spirit and Recovery

The human spirit is a remarkable force that drives individuals to overcome adversity, achieve great things, and plays a critical role in the recovery process. The intangible quality gives people the resilience to recover from setbacks and challenges and the courage to face the unknown with hope and optimism. When it comes to recovery, whether from physical or emotional trauma, injury, illness, addiction, neurological and mental health conditions or other challenges, spirit plays a critical role.

At its core, spirit is an expression of one's innate desire to thrive and grow. It is about seeking new experiences and opportunities, connecting with others, and being a part of something bigger than oneself. It is the source of motivation and creativity when facing adversity. When one experiences trauma or hardship, the spirit can be tested, but it is often in those moments that one also discovers their greatest strengths.

Recovery is a process that requires a tremendous amount of inner determination. The journey can be long and challenging. It can involve physical, emotional, and psychological obstacles. However, your spirit has an incredible capacity for healing and growth. With the right mindset, you can tap into your inner reserves of tenacity and character to overcome even the most challenging obstacles. We have been fortunate to witness this countless times throughout our work.

Perhaps one of the most significant ways in which the spirit plays a role in recovery is through the power of hope. Hope is a fundamental human emotion that gives one the valiant effort to face the unknown and to believe that better days are ahead. For individuals in recovery, hope can be a lifeline. It provides the motivation to keep going, even when the journey seems overwhelming.

You can overcome even the most daunting obstacles by tapping into your inner resources and surrounding yourself with support and compassion. When you do, you emerge stronger and wiser than ever before.

Accessing spirit goes beyond using a substance that induces the brain to briefly change chemically. Whether it's marijuana, alcohol, or another drug, these involve an outside element or approach to change the brain for a temporary transcendent experience. Evidence of the spiritual is found in the everyday feelings and experiences of the human journey. This can occur naturally, without opening a Pandora's box, by inducing distress on the brain for a short-lived experience, which can sometimes introduce long-term effects on your complex neuro-circuitry. Alcohol is often referred to as 'spirits' and is an in*toxic*ating substance to your brain. For your brain, there is no healthy amount of alcohol or drugs. Everything has long-term positive or negative consequences.

Self-Actualization and Spirit

> What one can be, one must be. This need we may call self-actualization. A musician must make music, an artist must paint, a poet must write if they are to be ultimately happy.
>
> - Abraham Maslow

Returning to Maslow's Hierarchy of Needs, the top of his pyramid is self-actualization. This is achieved with the realization that what's truly important is your creativity, intellect, and unique potential. Looking at George Vaillant's research, you can see that Maslow's hierarchy is similar to Vaillant's findings on spiritual evolution.

Self-actualization is not about material wealth or achieving the highest status. It's the internal drive to achieve a life that matters to you. Martin Seligman says that cultivating a life of experiences that matter leads to a life of meaning. It's seemingly less daunting to decide what matters to you than to determine what's meaningful or what your purpose is. If you say that freedom matters to you, then your actions will naturally draw you to live your life in a meaningful way that fulfills this need for you. On the other hand, if freedom matters to you as a core value, and you don't live a lifestyle in which you achieve it, then you risk being unfulfilled.

Self-actualization is about realizing your dreams, whether it's a career or personal life. It's about seeking what sparks your passion. Humans uniquely have the power of imagination, which is the inception to our dreams.

Self-actualization is the highest level of human needs. It's most commonly associated with acceptance of facts, lack of prejudice, problem-solving, morality, creativity, and spontaneity.

Dr. Marian Diamond—More on Enriched Environment

We already introduced neuroscientist Dr. Marian Diamond and her ground-breaking work in discovering neuroplasticity in the

1960s. We talked about how the first two things she discovered made for a robust brain: food and exercise. She also found that rat's brains flourished with:

- Newness
- Challenge
- Love

Newness can be defined as anything that is fresh to your brain, meaning that you have not learned it before. For example, when you learned how to tie your shoes, it was a new skill. When your brain learns a new skill, new neural pathways are formed. When you've mastered tying your shoes, your brain isn't getting the same benefit in terms of actual learning. Newness can be a new environment, a new skill, new language, new relationship, new career, a new hobby...you get the idea!

Challenge is also highly beneficial for your brain and can be deemed as doing something that pushes you beyond your comfort zone so long as this isn't so far out that it creates anxiety. This can be a physiological challenge at the gym by lifting greater weight. You can challenge your body with a nice hot sauna afterward to create Hormetic stress. Hormetic stress, or hormesis, is a controlled, acute stress that can trigger a healthy adaptive response. You can create challenges in a psychological sense, by choosing to embark on a new social experience. Or it could be something that challenges your beliefs and thoughts. It doesn't have to be a trip up Mount Everest. In fact, the brain responds very well to small daily challenges!

The last thing Dr. Diamond discovered that created a bigger, better brain was...***love***. She and her team discovered this in collaboration with European scientists. Their study of rats observed that the European rats had far greater longevity than the California rats. When they discussed care of the rats, Dr. Diamond learned that the other team took their rats out of their environments to hold them close to their chests and nuzzle them. The outcome of giving love to the rats increased their lifespan beyond anything the team in California had seen!

Returning to love, you'll recall that this was one of George Vaillant's seven key positive emotions shared earlier in this chapter. In Vaillant's book, *Spiritual Evolution*, he states, "Love is the shortest definition of spirituality I know."

Love and connection had been missing from Dr. Diamond's Experiments. It became crystal clear what a profound difference it made for the brain (and spirit) of the rat living an enriched life.

Learning Disorder or Creative Genius? The Gillian Lynne Story

Sir Ken Robinson wrote a book called *The Element*, based on a series of interviews with people on how they discovered their talent and how passion changes everything. Here is the story he shares about Gillian Lynne (1926–2018) in his own words in the famous TED Talk called *Do Schools Kill Creativity?* As we write this book, the video currently has over 23 million views.

Gillian Lynne was a legendary dancer and the choreographer of the wildly successful Broadway plays Cats and Phantom of the Opera.

When Gillian was in elementary school, she was hopeless, according to others. The school wrote to her parents, saying, "We think Gillian has a learning disorder." She couldn't concentrate; she was fidgeting. In modern times, they would most likely say she has ADHD. However, this was in the 1930s, and ADHD hadn't been created at this point. People weren't aware a condition like this existed.

Gillian went to see a specialist in an oak-paneled room. She was there with her mother, Mrs. Lynne. Gillian was led to a chair at the end of the room. She sat on her hands for 20 minutes while this man talked with her mother about all Gillian's problems at school. Her mother shared how she was disturbing people, her homework was always late, and so on; remembering, this is a young 8-year-old child.

In the end, the doctor went and sat next to Gillian. He said, "Gillian, I've listened to all these things that your mother has told me, and I need to speak to her privately." He went on to say, "Wait here and we'll be back. We won't be very long." The doctor left with her mother.

But as they went to leave the room, the doctor turned on the radio that was sitting on his desk. When they left the room, he said to Gillian's mother, just stand and watch her. The minute they left the room, Gillian was on her feet, moving to the music. They watched her for a few minutes. The doctor turned to her mother, and he said, "You know, Mrs. Lynne, Gillian isn't sick; she's a dancer. Take her to a dance school."

Sir Ken asked Gillian, "What happened?" Gillian replied, "She did, and I can't tell you how wonderful it was. We walked into this room, and it was filled with people like me; people who couldn't sit still, people who had to move to think."

They shared that it was filled with people who did ballet, tap, jazz, modern, and contemporary. Gillian eventually auditioned for the Royal Ballet School. She became a soloist and had a remarkable career at the Royal Ballet, eventually graduating from the Royal Ballet School. She went on to found her own company, the Gillian Lynne Dance Company and even met Andrew Lloyd Webber.

Gillian Lynne was responsible for some of history's most successful musical theatre productions. She delighted millions of audience members and was recognized as a world-class choreographer and director in television and live theatre. In 2018, the New London Theatre was officially renamed the Gillian Lynne Theatre.

It took an exceptional doctor's experience, wisdom, and creativity to recognize Ms. Lynne's gifts, even at a young age, and encourage the family to lean into her gifts and talents. This is the essence of positive psychology, a strengths-based approach to human development and Maslow's work in transcending through life.

Three Principles on Which Human Life Flourishes

Sir Ken Robinson's 2013 TED Talk, *How to Escape Education's Death Valley,* has currently had nearly 6.5 million views. In this talk, Sir Ken shares the three principles in which we flourish:

1. Human beings are naturally different and diverse as individuals
2. Curiosity, not compliance
3. Human life is inherently creative

Imagine what a wonderful world it could be if these principles were taught to all children – instead of teaching about bullying and competition to be the best at all costs. Imagine how the spirit might soar in this environment of flourishing principles.

Random Acts of Kindness (RAOK)

One of the most significant activities that our clients engaged in while enrolled in our program was Random Acts of Kindness Day. Each person got a small budget to purchase a costume at a local used clothing store and got to choose other accessories from our Tickle Trunk of items left by previous clients. The reason we dressed up in crazy costumes was that most people who attended our program typically had a paralyzing fear of being judged – especially in public. This was a pretty ingenious experiential therapy that helped people realize it was okay to be different and to stand out and be noticed – especially when it could bring a smile and joy to others. When everyone was outfitted, the coaches would take the group out to practice as many random acts of kindness as they could. Dave and Susan have fond memories of hearing the incredible tales of the magic and miracles that would always present themselves when the groups sought ways to spread the love.

One incredible story emerged from the group that came across a young woman whose car had quit; she was in tears because she was going to be late for a job interview. She was a single mom who had been out of work for a stretch of time and was frantic that she was going to miss this opportunity. Our quick-acting coach loaded her into the van, and they safely dropped her at her interview on time. He also knew a great mechanic who could fix her car and didn't charge her for it. They picked her up after the interview, and although we never found out if she got the job, the group was beyond proud of what they had made happen that day. The woman called our group 'angels.' We have hundreds of stories like this, and RAOK was always one of the most meaningful days for many.

Being of service and caring about others brings about a profound spiritual healing. On those days, our clients were superheroes dressed in strange duds, delivering joy and feeling like they made a difference in someone else's lives. That's powerful!

Random acts of kindness measurably activate brain regions associated with reward and empathy. This enhances mood, reduces stress, and promotes a calming sense of connection and wellbeing, which assures your brain that you're safe in this world.

We invite you to experience the effects of practicing kindness with intention and experience this magnificent change in your brain first-hand. Dressing up in costume is optional but highly recommended. It's loads of fun!

Chapter 9

Connections
The Fourth Principle

The opposite of addiction is not sobriety.
The opposite of addiction is human connection.

- Johann Hari

Family Bonds – Begin With Trust

When we began working with families, we intuitively knew that it was essential to have fully transparent conversations that included everyone in the family. It was one of many features that made our recovery program unique.

Many people who came to us to enroll in the recovery program were used to keeping secrets or telling some people one story and others a different story. This is called triangulation, and some people are masters at it. Triangulation can also be defined as manipulation due to the planning and intention of not fully disclosing.

For everyone to feel safe, openness is essential. From the get-go, we knew that truthful and transparent communication had to be part of the therapeutic plan for our clients to heal the past fully.

To begin the program, the client had to agree that everything they shared with anyone on our team was sharable for their best interests. For some people, this was new and challenging. For example, a young adult could be used to confiding in Mom and not talking with Dad. For long-term recovery, it's imperative to have everyone operating from the same place. In many cases, these clients had learned how to control connections by controlling communication from a young age.

At times, this concept of open sharing was way out of the comfort zone for the client's relationships. Yet, when we got to the place of honest and direct interactions, there was a freedom in the family that created a new bond, and we saw it again and again - it definitely brought them closer together.

To support people in unlocking their extraordinary, honest communication is paramount. Living from the truth and clear communication between all parties creates deeper and more meaningful connections.

Building on this, we created the acronym LOVE to help families thrive in their sacred connection:

L – Long-term
O – Ownership of
V – Values for
E – Everyone

Introducing this concept for the family to define their value system was much like a corporation with a mission statement. LOVE gave the family a starting point for new and rich connections.

We often found with families that there were competing ideas and values the family had to work through to get to the place of shared acceptance and agreement. Through our program, the family could develop a new creed by which to deal with conflict in a way that was respectful to and inclusive of all members. When you are totally heard within your own family, whatever your role, you feel connected to yourself as a result.

One of the roles of a Crisis and Recovery Coach is the neutral and safe axis that can facilitate essential conversations, leading to a new beginning. By doing so, the coach has the honor of witnessing a family become deeply connected. This is one of the most rewarding parts of the Recovery Coaches career.

The role of a Crisis & Recovery Coach is the neutral and safe axis that can facilitate essential conversations, leading to a new beginning.

The Emerging New Field of Social Neuroscience

Social Neuroscience is a field of study that combines neuroscience, psychology, and social sciences to explore how social interactions, relationships, and group dynamics impact the brain and behavior. It aims to understand the neural mechanisms underlying social behavior and the impact of social factors on the brain.

Social Neuroscience uses various methods, including brain imaging, and electrophysiology (the study of electrical properties) of biological and behavioral studies. Its purpose is to investigate how the brain processes and responds to social stimuli such as facial expressions, body language, and social cues. Researchers in this field also explore how social experiences shape the development of the brain and how brain activity is influenced by social context.

Social Neuroscience has provided insights into a range of social phenomena, including empathy, altruism, aggression, and social influence. It has also helped to advance understanding of social behavior, such as autism spectrum disorder and social anxiety.

One of the key findings of Social Neuroscience is that social interactions and relationships are *crucial* for developing and maintaining a healthy brain.

Social Neuroscience is an interdisciplinary field, and its findings have important implications for various areas, including psychology, sociology, economics, and public policy. As understanding of the neural mechanisms underlying social behavior continues to evolve, Social Neuroscience will play an increasingly critical role in shaping the understanding of human social interactions and relationships.

> Social interactions and relationships are crucial for the development and maintenance of a healthy brain… while social isolation and loneliness can have negative effects on the brain.

Being connected and in relationships are crucial for a healthy brain because of the impact on the neural circuits that underlie social behavior and emotions. Social experiences such as receiving affection, social support, and positive feedback can activate the brain's reward centers and trigger the release of feel-good chemicals like dopamine and oxytocin. These chemicals are known to enhance mood, reduce stress and anxiety, and promote social bonding.

In contrast, social isolation and loneliness can negatively affect the brain. Studies have shown that social isolation can lead to a range of physical and mental health problems, including addiction, depression, anxiety, cognitive decline, and an increased risk of mortality.

Research has shown that social interactions can also affect the structure and function of the brain. For example, studies have shown that the amygdala, a brain region involved in emotional processing, is larger in individuals with more social support. In contrast, the size of the amygdala is smaller in individuals who report feeling lonely or socially isolated. These findings suggest that social interactions can influence the development of brain structures critical for emotional regulation.

In addition, social interactions can also influence the activity of the brain's stress response system. Research has shown that social support can buffer the effects of stress on the brain and body. For example, social support has been shown to reduce the activity of the hypothalamic-pituitary-adrenal (HPA) axis, which is responsible for releasing stress hormones like cortisol. In contrast, social isolation can lead to increased activity of the HPA axis and higher levels of stress hormones in the body.

Furthermore, Social Neuroscience has highlighted the importance of social connection in promoting brain plasticity, the ability of the brain to adapt and change in response to new experiences. This means that social support can literally help to reshape the brain in ways that support recovery.

The Neuroscience of Human Connection

Human connections are fundamental to our emotional and physical wellbeing, and neuroscience has shed light on the underlying mechanisms that make these connections possible. Our brains are wired to form social connections for our very survival and to respond to social cues such as facial expressions, vocal intonations, and body language. These cues activate a network of brain regions known as the social brain, which includes the amygdala, the anterior cingulate cortex, the insula, and the prefrontal cortex.

The amygdala is essential in processing emotional information and is responsible for our ability to recognize and respond to the emotions of others. The anterior cingulate cortex is involved in empathy, social cognition, and decision-making processes related to social interactions. The insula is responsible for our ability to perceive and respond to physical sensations, including pain, touch, and temperature, and plays a crucial role in our experience of empathy. Finally, the prefrontal cortex is responsible for higher-order cognitive functions such as planning, decision-making, and social behavior.

By understanding that the brain drives social behavior, we can develop interventions and strategies to promote social connections that create deep, meaningful relationships. As we shared in Chapter

5, the Harvard Grant Study concluded that close relationships, more than money or fame, keep people genuinely happy throughout their lives.

What Isolation Does to the Brain

There's a reason why prisons use solitary confinement as the ultimate punishment.

> Loneliness isn't the physical absence of other people, it's the sense that you are not sharing anything that matters with anyone else.
>
> - Johann Hari

Isolation, whether self-imposed or forced, can have a profoundly negative impact on the brain and its functioning. The human brain is a highly social organ, and social interactions are crucial for maintaining its health. When we are isolated, our brains can undergo changes that can have negative consequences for our mental and physical health.

One of the most immediate effects of isolation on the brain is activating the stress response. When we are socially isolated, our brains perceive it as a threat to survival, and the stress response is triggered. This response can lead to increased levels of cortisol, a hormone that can have toxic effects on the brain and body when present at high levels for extended periods of time.

Isolation can also lead to changes in brain structure and function. Studies have shown that social isolation can result in decreased activity in the prefrontal cortex, a brain region responsible for decision-making, emotional regulation, and social behavior. This can lead to difficulty in regulating emotions and behaviors, as well as impairments in decision-making and problem-solving.

Overall, the effects of isolation on the brain are complex and multifaceted. Social interactions are essential for maintaining vibrant brain health, and prolonged isolation can have significant negative consequences. It is important to prioritize social connections; in fact, the research indicates that it is THE most important principle we should focus on and develop.

Johann Hari

Johann Hari is a writer and journalist who has written extensively on addiction and the importance of human connection in overcoming addiction. His research led him to state that the prevailing view of many is that addiction is a purely chemical and individual problem, which is incomplete and fails to address the root causes of addiction.

According to Hari, the opposite of addiction is not sobriety but rather human connection. In his phenomenal book *Lost Connections*, he cites studies showing that people who have strong social connections and meaningful relationships are less likely to develop addiction and are more likely to recover from it.

Johann Hari's work on addiction and human connection challenges the traditional understanding of addiction. Instead, he suggests that addiction is primarily a response to deeper emotional pain, trauma, and social disconnection.

Hari digs deep to discover that societal factors such as poverty, trauma, and lack of social support play a significant role in the development of addiction. He contends that people turn to drugs and other addictive behaviors to escape from this pain and to seek relief from feelings of loneliness, despair, and hopelessness. This mirrors Dr. Marian Diamond's discovery of diminished brain capacity while living in an impoverished environment.

He suggests that policies that criminalize drug use and punish drug users are unlikely to be effective in addressing addiction. Instead, a more compassionate and holistic approach is needed.

Hari's work highlights the importance of human connection in promoting eudaemonia (a contented state of being happy, healthy, and prosperous, and Dave's favorite word). It suggests that addressing social isolation and disconnection can play a critical role in preventing and overcoming addiction.

To address addiction prevention, Hari suggests that we need to focus on rebuilding social connections and communities. He highlights the importance of creating supportive environments where people can form meaningful relationships and feel a sense of belonging.

Hari's work has been influential in shifting the conversation around addiction, sparking a broader discussion on the critical role of human connection. His work also underscores the need for more comprehensive and compassionate approaches to addressing addiction, including providing access to mental health care, social services, and community-based support programs.

One of the primary challenges of traditional addiction recovery models is often the loss of social connections and support networks that can occur as a result of drug use and related behaviors. This can lead to feelings of loneliness, isolation, shame, and a lack of purpose, which can, in turn, contribute to relapse.

To address these challenges, recovery programs often focus on building social connections and supporting individuals in recovery. This can include group therapy, support groups, and other community-based gatherings that offer a sense of belonging and provide opportunities for meaningful social interactions. These groups and gatherings do not need to focus on recovery but rather on living the life you want. Then, they work collaboratively, supporting each other to achieve the life they choose, or as Dr. Diamond would call it – the enriched social environment.

Human beings are social creatures, and we thrive on connection and support from others. In recovery, having a strong support system can make a huge difference along with the brain-first focus. Whether it is family members, friends, a coach, or a supportive group, having people who understand and empathize with a person's challenges can be a powerful source of encouragement and motivation. To be clear, this support is not about allowing someone to stay in a victim helpless state of mind, but rather to live a life of achievement and personal meaning while contributing to others.

In the next chapter, Lifestyle, we will unveil the human equivalent of the enriched environment, and its enormous significance in the recovery field.

The Community Cure

The Community Cure by James Maskell, a healthcare entrepreneur, is a book that explores the concept of community-based healthcare and its potential to revolutionize the current healthcare system. It offers a compelling vision for the future of healthcare by bringing people together in groups so they don't feel isolated and alone.

Maskell is concerned that the current system primarily focuses on treating symptoms rather than addressing the root causes of health problems. More importantly, he shares that this standard is not sustainable. The medical community does not have the resources to provide individuals with the support they need to become healthy. Community and group-based approaches can offer a more holistic and effective solution.

His book presents several case studies and examples of successful community-based healthcare initiatives, such as group medical visits and health coaching programs. These programs involve patients coming together in a supportive and collaborative environment where they can learn from each other ***and*** receive personalized care from healthcare professionals.

Maskell also examines the role of technology in community-based healthcare and how it can facilitate communication and collaboration between patients and healthcare providers. He presents that by leveraging technology and other resources, community-based healthcare can provide high-quality care that is more accessible, affordable, and effective than the current redundant system.

Overall, *The Community Cure* offers a compelling vision for the future of healthcare, one rooted in community and focused on prevention and wellness rather than simply treating illness.

Much like Johann Hari, James Maskell advocates for a community-based approach to addiction treatment that recognizes the importance of social connections and support during recovery.

Maskell believes that addiction and recovery are complex and require a more holistic approach to treatment, as do we. He emphasizes that the current system of addiction treatment often focuses solely on managing the symptoms of addiction rather than addressing the underlying factors that create the problems in the first place. He believes in coaching programs where individuals can receive personalized care in a supportive and collaborative environment. Our internationally certified Crisis and Recovery Coaches can provide a resource within the community that lifts the burden from the medical model of care for those struggling with substance or behavioral habits.

Maskell emphasizes the importance of addressing the root causes of addiction, such as trauma, stress, and environmental factors, so people can have more effective and long-lasting support in their recovery journey.

One study that Maskell cites is the Phoenix Multisport program, which is a community-based program that emphasizes physical activity and social connection as key components of recovery. The participants experienced significantly lower rates of relapse and reported higher levels of social support and quality of life compared to those who did not participate in the program.

Cultural contexts are also an additional factor within the community and social framework. Batja Mesquita is a social psychologist known for researching emotional, cultural, and social relationships. One of her main areas of focus is how cultural contexts shape emotions and how they influence social interactions. Mesquita has examined how people from different cultures express and experience emotions and how these differences affect relationships with others.

Her work determined that people from cultures that prioritize and place high value on positive emotions such as happiness, may have difficulty understanding and relating to people from cultures that prioritize expressing more negative emotions, such as sadness or anger, and vice versa.

In a study published in Social Cognitive and Affective Neuroscience journal, Mesquita and her colleagues used electroencephalography (EEG) to investigate how cultural differences in emotional expressions affect neural processing of emotional stimuli. The study found that participants from different cultures showed differences in brain activity, suggesting that cultural diversity in emotional expression are linked to differences in neural processing of emotional information.

While her research does not focus exclusively on neuroscience, this study (and many more not mentioned here) demonstrates the value of understanding the complex interplay between culture, emotion, and the brain.

Biophilia—The Connection and Love of Nature in All Living Things

Perhaps the greatest gift of connection we can give to our brain circuitry is found in the forest, on the beach, on a mountain, at the park, with animals, or in your backyard.

Biophilia is the innate and genetically determined affinity or love for the natural world that humans have developed over the course of evolution. It is the idea that humans have a deep and intuitive connection to other living organisms and natural environments, believed to have arisen through millions of years of coexistence with nature.

The concept of biophilia suggests that humans have a fundamental need for nature and that contact with the natural world is essential for our health, wellbeing, and quality of life.

Research has shown that exposure to nature has numerous beneficial effects on the human brain, including:

1. Reducing stress and anxiety: Spending time in nature has been shown to lower cortisol levels, a hormone associated with stress. This can lead to reduced anxiety and an overall sense of calmness.
2. Boosting mood: Being in nature can help improve mood and increase happiness. Studies have found that just looking at nature scenes can lead to increased positive emotions.
3. Enhancing cognitive function: Exposure to nature has been shown to improve attention and memory and increase creativity and problem-solving abilities.
4. Promoting physical health: Spending time in nature can have physical health benefits, such as reducing

inflammation, lowering blood pressure, and improving immune function.

5. Restoring mental fatigue: Nature can provide a restorative effect, helping to replenish mental energy and reduce mental fatigue.

One recent study that provides evidence for the beneficial effects of nature on the brain was conducted by a team of researchers from the University of Illinois at Urbana-Champaign and published in the journal *NeuroImage* in 2021.

In this study, the researchers used functional MRI (fMRI) to investigate the neural effects of a 20-minute walk in a natural environment versus a busy urban environment. They found that participants who walked in the natural environment showed reduced neural activity in an area of the brain associated with rumination, which is a pattern of negative thinking that can contribute to depression and anxiety. In contrast, participants who walked in the urban environment showed no such reduction in neural activity.

This study provides evidence that exposure to nature can have specific and measurable effects on the brain and these effects may benefit mental health.

Through overwhelming research and our first-hand experience, it's clear that human connection with people and nature is vital for creating and sustaining neural networks that connect us to each other, the earth, and what matters most - to feel connected within ourselves.

Chapter 10

Lifestyle
The Fifth Principle

You are free to make whatever choice you want,
but you are not free from the consequences of the choice.

- Ezra Taft Benson (1899 – 1994)

Reverse Engineer Your Future

Most individuals create their future by looking at their present and past and consciously or unconsciously moving away from a pain point they ***don't*** want. Ask someone who is addicted to cigarettes what they want, and you'll probably hear, "I don't want to smoke." This way of thinking becomes your default. Saying, "I don't want to be broke" is not a plan to create prosperity, and you'll get more of what you're focusing on. This way of living is reactive to what's happened, so you've become stuck in these patterns.

To achieve true transformation, you must have a North Star to arrive at your destination. What is the future state that you *want* to live in? When you create your vision, you can reverse engineer how you arrive at that outcome and what actions you need to take to get there.

Sailors of old used the North Star to get them where they were headed, guiding them across the sea. They used their current location to navigate – where the journey started was irrelevant.

> Knowledge is power: You hear it all the time, but knowledge is not power. It's only potential power. It only becomes power when we apply it and use it.
>
> - Jim Kwik

Values Driven Life

When people are having difficulty completing goals, it's likely because they are fighting their desire for something new with their default mode to stay in their comfort zone. Your comfort zone is safe. It may not be great, and you may even loathe your present life, but it's predictable and requires less effort than changing. Fear bubbles up for many people when they think of embarking on a new life.

For example, when you open up a new Word document to begin to write, that document is set up with the font and the page layout. You can get as frustrated as you want, but your computer won't change the default mode until you set up a new default and save it so that you don't have to make changes again the next time you open Word.

Your brain has a default mode network of neuropathways running your habits because they're ingrained patterns within your neurocircuitry. Remember Hebb's Law – neurons that fire together wire together.

So, the question is, how do you override your default programming?

Get Uncomfortable

Challenging the fear of changing what is predictable, comfortable, and feels safe opens up a whole new world of what is possible. Humans have many different types of fear, which can be funneled down to three main categories: failing, looking silly, and not being liked. From an evolutionary point of view, your brain evolved to keep you safe. That is still your brain's primary role. We live in a modern world; however, your brain hardware is operating with outdated software.

Failing in the Stone Age meant you may put yourself in a risky situation and you may die. Looking silly – being different – meant you may not fit in with your tribe, and they may no longer trust you. Not being trusted and accepted meant the tribe could oust you, and you may die. Your brain has an excellent instinct; therefore, it is not advantageous to fail, look silly, or not be liked.

How do you override the default? By getting clear on what you personally value, aligning your choices with your values, and then embracing the unpleasantness of failing, looking silly, and perhaps not being liked. On the other side of these fears is your freedom.

Susan David, PhD, is a Harvard Medical School psychologist who studies the importance of people connecting with their values. Determining what's important to you must be viewed through the lens of what truly matters most to you. It's the beginning of your *why* to alter your status quo. Getting clear on values transcends simply being motivated to change.

For example, one of Dave's top values is autonomy because he unequivocally believes that he is responsible for his life, his choices, and his actions. His vocation has been to encourage others to embrace the power of freedom and choice and to live with extreme ownership. This is the polar opposite of the crushing emotional pain and spiritual prison of addictions.

One of Susan's top values is caring. One of the ways that this shows up is that she loves to bake for others. She says, "The world would be better with more home-baked cookies!" It's also self-care for her because she unwinds in the kitchen.

When you get clear on your values, it's your moral compass - actions align themselves with your personal core values. Decisions become easy through this lens. Inner turmoil (and addictions) surface when your beliefs and actions don't line up, and in many instances, this can lead to wanting to escape your fake life with numbing behaviors. These behaviors don't orient with your authentic truth, and that creates greater inner conflict.

Personal Values

Your Values are what you care about and consider the most important.

They are at the core of what you find meaningful in life.

Grab a pen. Review this list carefully. Consider what your top THREE values are and circle them or number them accordingly.

There is no right or wrong. This is your list.

- Reliability
- Trust
- Experimentation
- Responsibility
- Diversity
- Bravery
- Confidence
- Relationships
- Sensitivity
- Listening
- Simplicity
- Belonging
- Accuracy
- Curiosity
- Laughter
- Health
- Efficiency
- Caring
- Generosity
- Accountability
- Challenge
- Change
- Autonomy
- Community
- Cooperation
- Flexibility
- Adventure
- ________
- ________
- ________

Explore. Be Curious. And have some fun.

Source: Susan David, PhD, Harvard Medical School

Hedonism versus Eudaimonia

Hedonism is a philosophical concept that emphasizes the pursuit of pleasure and joy and the avoidance of pain as the primary goals of life. This could include engaging in activities such as indulging in unhealthy habits, prioritizing only enjoyable experiences, or seeking other forms of sensory pleasure. Hedonism is more about living in the moment impulsively and carries with it a greater possibility of regrets at the cost of long-term wellness and prosperity.

In a recovery context, hedonism might involve short-term strategies to alleviate the discomfort of stress, anxiety, or depression. Still, it could also come at a future cost if overindulgence in these pleasurable activities leads to neglect of other aspects of self-care, which risks jeopardizing your future.

Eudaemonia is a concept from ancient Greek philosophy that refers to a more profound and enduring sense of wellbeing and flourishing. Unlike hedonism, eudaimonia is not solely focused on momentary pleasure but on living a meaningful and purposeful life. Eudaemonia involves personal growth, self-actualization, and the realization of one's full potential.

In the context of a recovery lifestyle, eudaimonia would emphasize and carefully consider activities that foster a long-term thriving and authentic life of meaning.

Your Future is Lead by Your Mindset

Several years ago, we had a client in our recovery program (whom we will call Mike). Mike, a divorced father of two boys, worked as a tradesperson and had seniority at the company he worked for. He made enough income to provide the means for a comfortable life, a lovely home, some fun toys, a holiday once or twice a year, plus enough for savings.

When his marriage dissolved, he only saw his children every other week, and he became quite sad. He was already a cigarette smoker, began to drink more than he wanted to, and through some new acquaintances, he started using cocaine. His party lifestyle was rapidly becoming a big problem that was affecting his work performance and job security, his relationship with his sons and their mom, and his overall wellbeing was declining at high speed.

> If a young person is diagnosed with a mental health disorder, are their metabolic needs being met? Are their sleep needs being met? Are their exercise needs being met? Are their nutritional needs being met? Because if those needs aren't met then the response of anxiety and depression is not a disorder that's order.
>
> - David Bidler, How Changing Your Lifestyle Can Fix Your Mental Health
>
> - Dr Rangan Chatterjee's Podcast, Feel Better, Live More, ep. #408

Mike was suspended from work with a compassionate boundary to seek help quickly, and that's how he found Emergo. When Mike arrived, he was very thin and fragile with dark circles under his eyes, had a tough time sitting still, and yet was exhausted to the core.

After being with us for about a week, Mike was looking and feeling much healthier, and his energy was definitely increasing without the toxic brain substances he had been using. He was no longer jittery, laughing more, and feeling proud that he was diving into and loved learning about how his brain function and his behaviors were connected. He was feeling hopeful that he could recover his life – and was actually feeling better than he had in years.

It was July, and it was cherry season. One day, we were all enjoying the delicious taste of summer fruit, and Mike said he loved cherries – they were his favorite fruit. But then he went on to say that while he was grateful to have organic cherries and how incredible they tasted, there was no way that he could possibly afford to eat them at home because they were too expensive for his food budget.

One of the coaches asked him how much cigarettes, alcohol, and cocaine cost. In an instant, it was like a lightbulb went on for Mike, and in that moment, he had a complete mindset shift about his true priorities and values. And he had a good belly laugh at his silly excuse.

Henry Ford said it best, *"Whether you think you can or think you can't, you're right."*

Your beliefs make a profound difference in how you live your life. For Mike, the belief that fresh organic fruit was too expensive was preposterous when considering the cigarettes, alcohol, and cocaine he was spending his money on while destroying every part of his life and everything that mattered.

Mike's story is an easy example of how you can live with ideas and beliefs that prevent you from achieving what you want.

In the previous chapters, we have shared many brain-healthy lifestyle recommendations. Still, none of these will matter if you have an overarching belief or stuck mindset that will sabotage whatever upgrades you want.

Renowned psychologist Carol Dweck has devoted her life to studying mindset and how your brain can restructure and work to help you solve problems rather than giving up and reliving the same patterns. In 2006, she literally wrote the book on mindset called *Mindset: The New Psychology of Success*. Her studies have launched thousands of other researchers to plunge into this human superpower deeply. What she uncovered about the power of the mind is used by elite coaches, athletes, and highly successful individuals.

Dr. Dweck says there are two types of mindsets: the *growth mindset* and the *fixed mindset*. When you have a growth mindset, you believe you can gain the knowledge and skills necessary to succeed, making every challenge an opportunity for expansion. The opposite is a fixed mindset, and the implication is that if you don't already have the skills or intelligence to complete the task, or you believe that the problem is not your fault and out of your control, there is no chance of succeeding, so why even bother to try.

When you flip the switch on thinking that effort and difficulty are painful, with the belief that effort and difficulty are necessary precursors to your growth – your mind shifts to finding solutions and enjoys the process. When you are presented with a challenge that is hard and requires you to do something you haven't done before, simply saying, "I can't do it YET", (instead of I can't do it) sets your brain on a creative mission to find out how to achieve it.

With this one word, *yet*, you can actually rewire the neuro-connections in your brain. When you accept the challenge to grow beyond your limiting beliefs, you upgrade your lifestyle one neuropathway at a time.

When Quincy Jones, whose musical career has spanned more than 70 years, was asked to talk about some of the problems he has incurred in his lifetime, he said, "I don't have problems; I have puzzles." That's a growth mindset statement that engages the brain to find answers.

This is not about willpower. If you think you've failed in the past because you lack willpower, we have great news for you. You don't need willpower. You need to cultivate a growth mindset that fully embraces a brain-healthy lifestyle.

You may have a belief that change is hard. You may have been told that quitting substances or giving up self-sabotaging habits is difficult. What's really hard is living in lies, feeling disappointed in yourself, and letting down the people who love and care about you – over and over again. What's hard is breaking promises and trust. What's hard is seeing your life slip by. What's hard is doing things that you regret, and not living up to your potential. What's hard is being dependent on things outside of yourself for comfort. What's hard is drifting.

What's easy is having robust physical and mind health, control of your life, honesty, independence, fulfillment, self-respect, time freedom (when you're not thinking about your next drink, cigarette, or Instagram scroll) and your wealth to share as you wish.

Extrinsic Motivation versus Intrinsic Inspiration

People don't resist change – they resist being changed. Whenever you perceive that you have been forced to adopt a new lifestyle (told you must by a boss, physician, authority, or a family member), any changes are likely to be short-lived because this is extrinsic or coming from an outside influence. Perhaps you feel resentment, and with that emotion as the catalyst, nothing will stick because you're not driving the change. "I should" is not "I will".

Being motivated to revise your life is usually initiated by a sudden awareness that if you don't do things differently, there could be a negative consequence. This is also likely to be short-lived and when the crisis has passed, its more likely that you'll slip back into old patterns. Motivation is also extrinsic, therefore, there's a much greater chance that it's short-term.

A genuine and sustained overhaul of your life occurs within your mind first. This is intrinsic – initiated within you. It's done with intention and inspiration that you can get through the adversity that will appear on the journey to rebuild and remake yourself. You meet these challenges with resolve and confidence that you have a growth mindset no matter what, and you'll solve whatever *puzzle* comes your way. You're ready to rewrite your past pain story into your hero's journey.

Tiny Habits and Your Brain

BJ Fogg is a charismatic researcher and author focusing on behavior change and habit formation. He has written extensively on the topic of *Tiny Habits*. These tiny, easy-to-implement habits can lead to incredible, meaningful behavior changes. Fogg's approach to behavior change is based on his analysis of how the brain works and how habits are formed. Fogg's research has shown that the brain responds best to small, incremental changes that are linked to positive emotions and rewards.

According to Fogg, the brain is wired to respond to rewards by seeking pleasure and avoiding pain. He notes that habits are formed when behaviors are consistently linked to rewards. In order to create new habits, Fogg suggests identifying small behaviors that can be easily incorporated into existing daily routines and then can be linked to a positive emotion or reward.

Note that Fogg emphasizes that habits are formed when behaviors are linked to ***rewards***, not drudgery or punishment. Not self-deprecating nagging self-talk. If you've self-sabotaged your efforts in the past, maybe you want to take a look at instilling a reward to forge new circuitry.

Professor Fogg made the incredible connection that building new habits around activities you already do regularly, is easier and more successful than inserting a new habit not connected to an existing one. Example – while you're brushing your teeth in the morning, do squats for two minutes. When you've finished the workout, celebrate with a high-five in the mirror or a self-congratulatory whoop or dance for your effort. Think of professional athletes after they score.

Fogg suggests starting with tiny habits such as flossing one tooth after brushing (you already have the habit of brushing). Another example is doing two push-ups after waking up in the morning (something you do every day). These tiny habits are easy to do and can be completed in less than 30 seconds, and they can still provide a sense of accomplishment and a positive feeling of progress. All of a sudden you are the person who does push-ups and flosses your teeth! It's not the number of push-ups or the teeth flossed, it's developing a tiny new habit that's sustainable. Have an apple on your desk instead of an unhealthy snack.

As soon as you finish the tiny habit—in the example above, it would be flossing one tooth, doing two push-ups, or eating the apple—you MUST celebrate the achievement in the moment it is completed. This is the reward the brain needs to know that this is a habit worth doing again!

Think about when children are small. We'll use the example of tying their shoes to illustrate how new neural connections are formed in the brain. What do the adults do when a child is learning a new skill? They cheer and become very animated when the child applies effort. The child continues to work hard because they are enjoying the praise and championing of their efforts – the reward. This celebration encourages kids to keep doing the task, eventually leading one day to successfully tying the shoes (new neural connections have begun).

Over time, Fogg suggests gradually increasing the difficulty of the tiny habits as they become more ingrained. Individuals can create new habits and achieve meaningful behavior change by consistently linking small behaviors to rewards.

Fogg's research is grounded in the concept of *behavior design*, which involves identifying the specific behaviors that individuals want to change, and designing strategies to help them create new habits. According to Fogg, the key to successful behavior design is to focus on tiny habits that are easy to do and that can be consistently linked to a positive emotion or reward.

He also recommends using prompts for the new habit that you want to engage with, whether that's sticky notes (Susan's go-to), setting up your running shoes to be the first thing you see when you wake up, putting a dumbbell in your bathroom, or an alarm on your phone. The easier it is, the better your chance of doing it consistently. Relying on willpower and memory isn't likely to work.

In this same line of thinking, make the habits that you no longer want, very difficult and challenging. If it's a certain food you can't resist, don't have it in your home. If it's TV that you want to reduce, hide the remote controls in a different room, or unplug the TV so you'll have to wait for it to reset. If it's alcohol, don't drive the route that takes you to your favorite liquor store, arrange to do other things with friends rather than go for a drink, and set up your environments with the things you do want. Get creative, as you have already discovered your brain loves that!

Creating your new life is all about brainpower, not willpower.

NOT a Relapse Plan

When you enter a destination into your device, it will provide you with the optional routes to arrive where you want to go. It would seem silly to enter in a target that you don't want. This is like driving your car by looking in the review mirror. Creating an actual intention for a relapse plan plants seeds of doubt in your brain, and you've already planned for your failure. In fact, you may have been told in the past that it's an essential part of your recovery.

Instead, fill your life with people you find engaging, things you want to consume that increase your energy, and activities that you want to do. Set up your environments to support this rousing plan. And using the driving your car analogy – look in front of you!

The opposite of addiction is living well. Focusing on a vibrant life of wellbeing and creating a robust support plan is the opposite of a relapse plan. Words have power, they become the map for how we think.

Crafting Your Personal Enriched Environment

Throughout these pages, we have provided a blueprint for what an enriched environment looks like. Focusing on the first four principles of Actualized Recovery will give you a solid foundation that drives transformation. Physiology, Psychology, Spirit, and Connection are the vital elements that will serve as the starting point for your wellbeing, autonomy, and longevity.

Doing something 100% is a heck of a lot easier than 99%.

When you commit FULLY to anything, the shift becomes easier, and transitions happen much faster. If you are on a diet and decide to have a cheat meal or a cheat snack, that one deviation can have a ripple effect that actually makes your healthy lifestyle goal harder; it puts your goal in greater jeopardy. You also have this voice going off in your head that you have to push away or ignore. That voice can be quite cunning and will work to find your weak spots....come on you deserve it; it's been an extra stressful time. Or maybe the excuse of a celebration sets off that inner voice. And knowing you are okay with some cheat days....why not today? And so goes the battle.

Moderation rarely works for anyone, and if you have an addiction of any kind, moderation is not the solution – your brain doesn't work that way; it's an all-in or all-out monogamous kind of organ! What does work? A commitment. A complete commitment to what you want. Get clear and use the knowledge to better understand the cascading impact of 99%. A 100% commitment is like taking a huge cannonball in the deep end of the pool. If you want a different outcome, you need to take a different action, which means abstinence. If you have an alcohol dependence, drinking zero alcohol – including the 'non-alcoholic' versions that mimic your old vices – is the only way to fully overcome it and move forward because you have established neuropathways associated with drinking. Reinforcing negative or self-harming neural pathways (meeting at the bar and swearing you'll only drink water) is like playing Russian Roulette. If your slippery slope is cheese, allowing yourself to binge occasionally will keep it top of mind, and your cravings will continue, particularly if you treat cheese like a reward.

Bill (not his real name) was a former drinker and heavy gambler. The wreckage his addictions caused was brutal. He lost his business. Lost his family. Lost the family home. Mountains of debt. He developed mental and physical illnesses and had almost given up hope that he could turn his life around.

Amazingly, five years go by, and Bill has not had a drink, no drugs, and the biggest win - zero gambling, including even buying lotto tickets. He has begun to rebuild his life with a new relationship, restored his income, has a successful new business, and has regained his health and happiness. So, he decided that he would go to Las Vegas for his five-year celebration to honor his diligent work and new lifestyle. Yup, Vegas! And why not? He 'knows' he's got it all under control. Flights, hotels, and meals are cheap. The weather is great. Golfing is fantastic. And he can take in some shows. Bill's arrogance defends this as the best location to go because he says he can test himself and prove that he has this all dialed in. "I've got this."

We all know this is likely a brutal idea. This is not a stellar decision for so many reasons. Going to Vegas is a decision of ego, a careless and reckless risk. And why? What for?

Vegas trips were part of his old lifestyle, and he remembers the fun and wants to re-live that excitement minus the pain. Here's why it's not the best plan...because the moment his brain hears the slots, sees the tables and the bright lights, and he's offered multiple free drinks, his brain will instantly awaken those old neural pathways...and now he has to over-ride the compulsion to drink and gamble again, in an environment that is all about drinking and gambling! He is going to have to rely on willpower over and over and over again to say no. Not once but hundreds of times during his 'vacation'.

We share this story to illustrate what happens when we think that we can reintroduce old destructive habits and lose focus on *what we want*. Remember, it's not about willpower – overcoming addiction and behaviors is about brain power.

A 100% commitment to a new lifestyle would mean a trip to Florida, fishing in Minnesota, or hiking in the Rocky Mountains—a lot easier to maintain the life you want and thrive. A lot easier!

The question to ask is, when do you put yourself at anything less than 100%? Do you meet old friends at your favorite bar? Do you skip that yoga session you booked and scroll through social media? Do you buy a couple of pints of your favorite Häagen-Dazs ice cream at the store and bring it home? Do you grab your phone to check your favorite team's odds for tonight's big game, promising yourself you won't place a bet?

There is a wonderful and very popular band, *For King and Country.* If you haven't had the pleasure of hearing their music, check 'em out. Their music is fantastic and very inspirational. The lead members are two brothers, Luke and Joel. They were born in Australia, and their family moved to Nashville when they were young. To illustrate the above story, we have included an article from Billboard (billboard.com) published on October 8, 2018, addressing the value and importance of their hit song *Burn the Ships*.

The title track was inspired by Luke's wife Courtney battling addiction. The couple has three sons, and during her second pregnancy doctors prescribed an anti-nausea medicine to help Courtney with debilitating morning sickness. During the pregnancy, they continued to increase her dosage. "I was in Austin, TX for a show," Luke recalls. "Courtney calls me and said, 'Hey I need you to come home.' I said, 'Okay what's going on?' She said, 'I can't stop taking these pills. We've got to deal with this.'"

Luke returned immediately, took his wife to a psychiatric facility and doctors placed Courtney in a treatment program. Luke dropped her off every morning at 9am and picked her 2pm. "I was at home one day and she had a bottle of pills in her hand. I was like, 'What do you have the bottle of pills for?'" he recalls. "She said, 'Luke I need to flush these pills because these pills represent so much guilt and shame in my life. I don't want to be consumed by my past anymore. I want to move into a new day and to what's before me.'"

The album title came from that moment combined with an old history lesson. "I read a story about an explorer going to a new land. When he arrived on the shore, he calls everybody off of the ships and said, 'Hey let's go explore this land and see what there is to be seen,'" Luke explains. "All the men were terrified of going into the unknown and he realized that even those boats were grimy, stinky and small, they wanted to stay on the boats because it was familiar. The next day he calls them out again and when all the sailors were on land, he gives the command to burn the ships because he said, 'We're not going to retreat. We're going to move forward in our lives.' The flushing of the pills was the burning of the ships for my wife and for us to step into a new world, a new day. That was four years ago now. My wife said, 'You need to go share this story with people because there's so many people that are bound by things in their past. I don't want people to live like that. I want my story to be an encouragement to help them spread their wings.'"

Source: FOR KING AND COUNTRY ON THE STRUGGLES THAT INFORMED 'BURN THE SHIPS,' THEIR 'MOST MATURE RECORD' YET, by Deborah Evans Price, Billboard.com, 10/8/2018

Link – Article: https://www.billboard.com/music/rock/for-king-country-burn-the-ships-interview-8478875/

Link – Official Music Video (YouTube): https://www.youtube.com/watch?v=pOVrOuKVBuY

This story is to highlight that when you want a new beginning, it is essential to burn the ships. Of course, you don't have to; this is your choice. But the danger is always knowing and always having a way to turn back or go back.

Practicing and implementing the steps and principles of Actualized Recovery is your roadmap to a brighter, more vibrant future. It is vital to focus on your future and what you want.

You can certainly look at what you *don't* get to have. Many people do, and it's a prelude to failure. When you focus on what you do have, and you're grateful for everything, these gifts and this energy ripple throughout every part of your mind and instead of feeling deprived, you feel grateful.

What can you do today? Do you have alcohol or drugs you want to flush? What relationship(s) no longer serve you? What negative lifestyle choices need to go? Pick one thing right now and take action. It can be small or large, but pick one thing and take decisive action. Because 100% ALL-IN is a lot easier than 99%. Remember, 'Burn The Ships.'

Making Decisions Using 10-10-10

10-10-10 is a decision-making framework designed to help people gain clarity and make better choices in their personal and professional lives. Coined by Suzy Welch, a bestselling author and business journalist, the concept centers around considering the consequences of a decision in three different time frames: 10 minutes, 10 months, and 10 years.

The first step, the *10-minutes* perspective, encourages you to assess the immediate impact of your decision. It prompts you to consider how you would feel in the next few minutes or hours after making a choice. This short-term perspective is useful for addressing immediate concerns and emotions.

The second step, the *10-month* perspective, encourages you to project how your decision might unfold over the next several months. This medium-term view helps identify potential challenges and opportunities that may arise as a result of the decision.

The final step, the *10-year* perspective, pushes you to contemplate the long-term implications of a choice. By considering the consequences a decade into the future, you can evaluate the alignment of the decision with your values, goals, and aspirations.

The 10-10-10 framework fits beautifully with Viktor Frankl's choice theory. It's the gap to consider the possible outcomes of your decision through the lens of immediate, mid-range, and long-term consequences that can provide incredible and immediate clarity. Although you can't know for certain, utilizing this strategy usually creates an obviousness in the best direction. What's great is that it literally takes seconds to run through it in your mind, and once you make the decision, there is a certainty that settles and makes it easy to take the next steps.

We've taught this concept to hundreds of people over the years, and the feedback has always been enthusiastic. Dave and Susan will often ask each other, "10-10-10" for small or large decisions they need to make, and it works every time!

Using 10-10-10 can prevent hasty and emotionally driven decisions that may lead to regret in the long run. It allows us to think more strategically and holistically, promoting a balanced approach to decision-making. The process enables us to prioritize our choices based on our long-term vision while addressing immediate needs and concerns.

Big Rocks

Instead of telling you how to design your life, we'd rather guide you to create the best possible opportunity for you to thrive by making these lifestyle priorities through a brain-first lens. We used to do an experiential project with clients that involved them finding different sizes of rocks. They would name these rocks as the priorities that they wanted to focus on in their lives. We would provide a large clear glass container and sand. Step one of this project was to fill the glass container to the top with sand.

Step two was to take the rocks that they chose and identified with their priorities and do their very best to force those rocks as far into the container as they could. It was always messy and usually quite frustrating because no one could get their rocks very far.

Step three was to empty the container, place the rocks in first, and then add the sand. Adding the stones first was much easier and far more effective.

Once you choose your biggest rocks, add them to your schedule first and then let the rest of your day fill the space around them – like the sand around the rocks.

Here are some ideas for your biggest rocks:

1. Deep, meaningful relationships (family, friends, career)
2. Fun/play
3. Building prosperity
4. Generosity and kindness
5. Nourishment and hydration
6. Brain and liver detoxification
7. Sleep and restoration of energy

8. Spiritual development – knowing thyself and practicing faith
9. Movement to build and keep strength, flexibility, endurance, and balance
10. Challenge – building resilience, self-trust, and self-esteem
11. Newness – learning new things to keep you and your brain from getting old

Build Your Vision and Reverse Engineer

Leveraging what you've learned about Actualized Recovery:

Step 1: Imagine what you truly want. Write it all out, or create a vision board.
Step 2: Get clear on *why* you want each of these things, one by one.
Step 3: What value and meaning does each of these bring to your life?
Step 4: Decide the priorities to *start* doing, and what you need to *stop* doing to begin your quest.

If you feel that you are ready to map out your Actualized Recovery roadmap, that we've shared enough tools for you to construct the plan, and you're inspired to begin your quest toward wellbeing, we wish you much joy and success!!

If you'd like some support, but still want to work on your own, you can join our community in our Actualized Recovery Tribe, and you can enroll in our self-directed on-line course to be guided while maintaining the freedom to work on your own timeline.

If you feel that you want a partnership to co-create your Actualized Recovery plan, connect with us and we'd be honored to put you in touch with one of our certified Crisis & Recovery Coaches, who know precisely how to lead you through this process by profoundly listening and then guiding and colaberating with you. Transformation works best when you have accountability, especially with a trained and certified Crisis & Recovery Coach who has taken many people on this journey.

If you're ready to create a career in lifting others while cementing your new lifestyle, you may want to join us to train and become an Internationally Certified Crisis & Recovery Coach. There is no better way to make a massive impact and create greater freedom in your life. You may be the light that someone is waiting for.

We sincerely hope that we have opened your heart and brain to possibilities that you may not have considered and that you can take from this book what excites and inspires you to implement *tiny habits* into your life that will create a massive shift for you over time. Like compounding interest – the growth can happen very quickly.

We are so grateful that you've invested your resources of time, energy, and money to read or listen to our book, and we thank you. We are delighted for you to harness the power of your brain and *Unlock Your Extraordinary.*

About the Author

Dave Kenney

Picture a nine-year-old grappling with the shame and defeat of failing grade four.

Now, envision him a year later, at age ten, failing grade four, again, for the second time.

Throughout his school years, Dave put forth his best effort, but success was elusive.

Then, in high school, his parents uncovered that Dave had a learning or brain dysfunction. The issue wasn't a lack of effort but a neurological hurdle. With the right interventions, a new path unfolded before him, one where learning and thriving became possible.

This pivotal experience profoundly shaped Dave's beliefs and life's mission. He holds a firm conviction that no one sets out to fail and that within each individual lies an inherent greatness, a unique potential to make a meaningful impact in the world.

The Actualized Recovery methodology and the authoring of this book are living proof of his belief. They stand as a testament to the idea that everyone, regardless of their struggles, can overcome obstacles and realize their dreams.

It is Dave's fervent hope that this book serves as a beacon of inspiration and a source of profound knowledge, empowering readers to embark on their own transformative journey. He dreams that everyone who delves into these pages emerges with the courage and insight to write their own extraordinary tale of comeback and victory.

About the Author

Susan Kenney

Susan's journey as a writer began at the tender age of 10, perched in front of her parents' electric typewriter. Her early ambition was to craft a book filled with magic and hope for children who needed it most.

From her earliest memories, Susan's greatest joy has always been reading. The Nancy Drew series was a particular favorite. She often frustrated her mother because she would read books cover to cover within hours.

Susan's early years were shaped by her older sister, Linda Marie, whose life was marked by brain damage, turning even the simplest tasks into monumental challenges. This first-hand experience with the profound limitations of a compromised brain forged in Susan an unwavering appreciation and intricate understanding of the brain's immense power. She is committed to leading others to live a brain-first healthy lifestyle.

She is dedicated to unlocking the transformative power that comes from valuing this essential organ, which influences every facet and the overall quality of life.

In her professional life, Susan serves as the Chief Research Officer at Emergo Academy. Her knack for grasping and teaching new information has even earned her the playful nickname of 'Dave's walking Soogle'. Devouring non-fiction is, without a doubt, her superpower!

Susan's favorite hobby is exploring and tweaking recipes.

Authoring a book has been a lifelong aspiration. Seeing it come to fruition is truly a dream come true.

Appreciation and Gratitude

The authors extend our heartfelt appreciation and profound gratitude to the myriad of individuals who have enriched and supported us throughout this remarkable journey.

Our deepest thanks go to our three children, who have supported us to devote our energies to helping others.

We are immensely grateful to our teachers and mentors, whose wisdom and guidance have been invaluable. Their lessons have been a guiding light in our endeavors.

To our clients and their families—your trust and faith have been a source of endless inspiration. It has been an honor to be part of your journey.

We owe a special debt of gratitude to the over 100 Crisis & Recovery Coaches, chefs, and health and therapeutic professionals. Your dedication and compassion were the lifeblood that realized our dream every day for the past twelve years. Your commitment to making the world a better place has been transformative.

Our acknowledgments would be incomplete without mentioning the experts who have dedicated their lives to their crafts. Your wisdom and creativity have been pivotal in shaping the content of this book. Standing on your shoulders, we have reached new heights.

Lastly, to our three English Golden Retrievers – Turk, Maslow, and Gracie – thank you for the love, laughter, and emotional healing you've provided to so many, ourselves included. Your presence has been a source of joy and comfort on this journey.

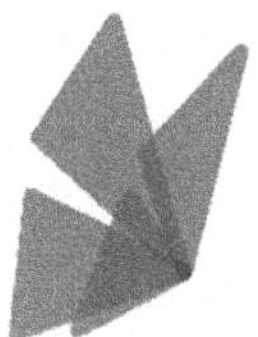

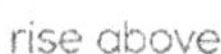

Emergo Academy

Your Online Recovery Tribe

Emergo Academy shines as a beacon of innovation and hope in recovery and personal transformation. More than a community, we are a movement dedicated to guiding individuals from their struggles and pain to a vibrant, fulfilling life.

As this book highlights, our approach transcends dependency, emphasizing overall wellbeing and flourishing. By embracing a brain-first approach and harmonizing the principles of physiology, psychology, spirit, connections, and lifestyle, you embark on a quest for profound and lasting personal transformation.

At Emergo Academy, we're not only about personal recovery; we also shape future leaders in the field of recovery. Our internationally certified coaching programs are meticulously crafted to develop skilled, empathetic Crisis & Recovery Coach Warriors prepared to inspire and orchestrate heroic comeback stories.

Whether focused on your recovery and wellbeing or aspiring to mentor and coach others, our programs offer a tailored blueprint for heroic impact and epic freedom.

Now more than ever, people need new tools and support to rise above

SCAN HERE

https://www.emergoacademy.com

the challenges in their lives and emerge as the most optimized, balanced, and empowered versions of themselves. This is what you will find at Emergo Academy.

We heartfeltly believe everyone has an awe-inspiring comeback story waiting to be lived.

So, join us and Unlock Your Extraordinary!

Notes

www.ingramcontent.com/pod-product-compliance
Lightning Source LLC
Chambersburg PA
CBHW052112030426
42335CB00025B/2949

* 9 7 8 1 9 2 3 1 2 3 6 4 9 *